Ten Doctors that Heal Mental Disease Naturally...

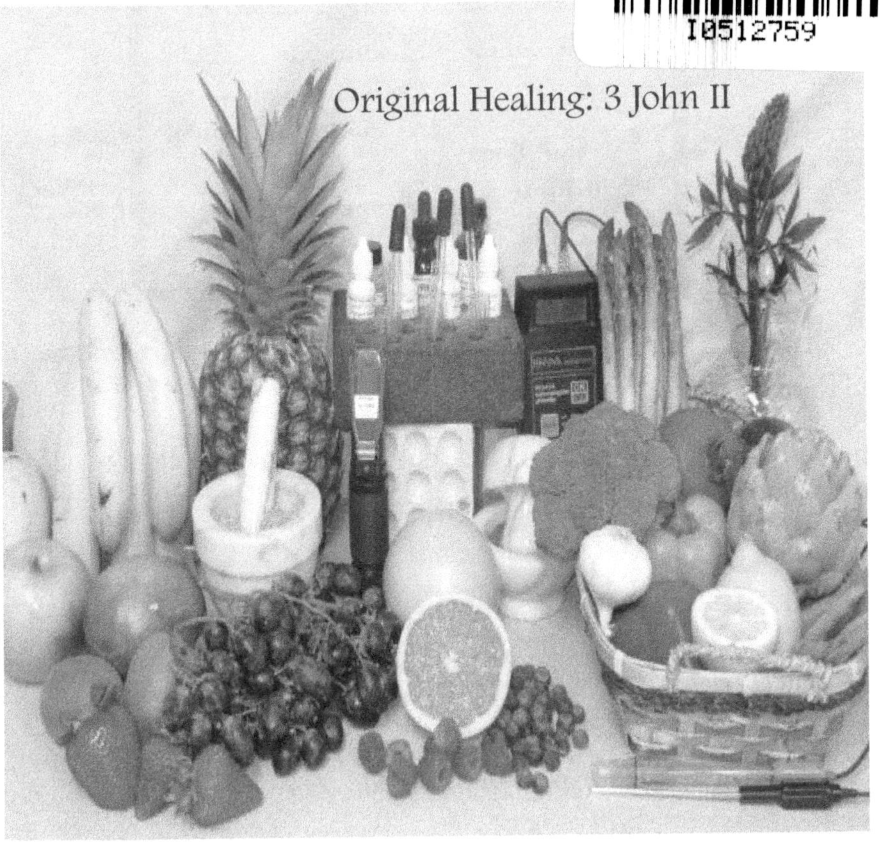

Original Healing: 3 John II

A Positive Thought!

Rick L. Lee, N.D., D.D.
Missionary Health Restoration Practitioner

The Ten Doctors

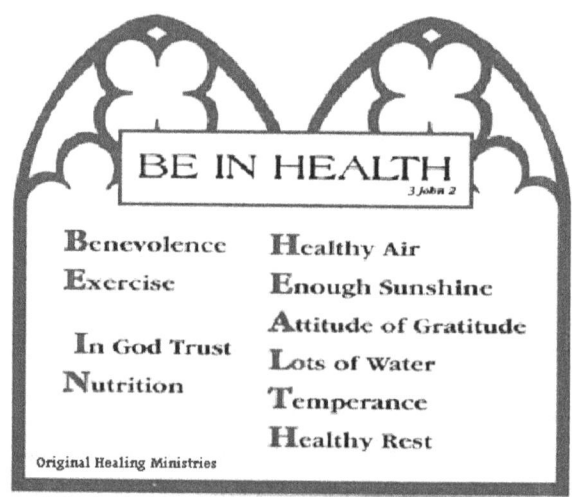

A Positive Thought

No rights reserved. All parts of this publication may be reproduced or utilized without written permission from the Author.

Editor: Rick L. Lee
      Wilda V. Lee

Printed in the United States of America

Second Edition March, 2019
The information in this book is for educational purposes only and is not recommended as a means of diagnosing or treating an illness. All, matters concerning physical and mental health should be supervised by a Health Restoration Practitioner knowledgeable in God's true methods of health restoration. Neither the publisher nor author directly or indirectly give medical advice, nor do they prescribe
Allopathic drugs. The author, editors, or publisher do not accept any responsibility for those who choose to treat themselves.

Other books by Rick L. Lee, N.D.
- Exalting the Standard of Righteousness
- No Healing Medicines (based on Jeremiah 30:13, 46:11).

TABLE OF CONTENTS

Be In Health	2
Table of Contents	3
Dedication	4
Introduction	5
Unintended Consequences	6
About the Author & Personal Experience	8
The Church of Modern Medicine	16
Chapter I: The Battle Field Is the Mind	17
Chapter II: His Servant ye are to whom ye obey	26
Chapter III: Psychiatry, God's Blessing or Man's Curse	28
• Diagnostic & Statistical Manuel (DSM)	31
• Diagnostic & Statistical Manuel II (DSM II)	33
• Diagnostic & Statistical Manuel III (DSM III)	34
Chapter IV: Poor Mental Health A Nutritional Deficiency?	36
Chapter V: Brain Chemicals	45
Chapter VI: The Food $ Drug Administration (FDA)	49
Chapter VII: 5-HTP and Depression	55
Chapter VIII: Dr. Sunshine	60
Chapter IX: Dr. Exercise and Dr. Water	61
Chapter X: Dr. Fresh Air	64
Chapter XI: Dr. Rest	66
Chapter XII: Dr. Godly Trust	67
Chapter XIII: True and false Systems of Mind Cure	70
Chapter XIIII: Make a New You: John 3:3	81
Chapter XV: What You can do to Strengthen Your Will	82
Chapter XVI: The Body Temple	93
Chapter XVII: God Heals Mental Diseases Naturally	105
Chapter XVIII: Herbs in the Laboratory	107
Chapter XIX: Rigorous Herbal Clinical Trials	110
Chapter XX: Dr. Hoffer's Natural Schizophrenia Protocol	112
Chapter XXI: Quotes from Famous Historical Vegetarians	118
Chapter XXII: Case Studies	121
Chapter XXIII: Safety of Natural vs. Synthetic Drugs	126
Chapter XXIV: School Shooting Linked to Synthetic Drugs	129

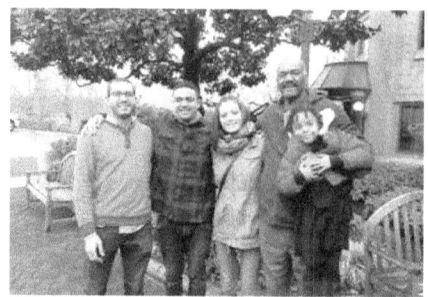

Dedications:

To my four thriving Children who by God's grace have matured and have become producers in society that I love very much. To my failed relationships whether life partner, teammate, or someone that our lives intersected, forgive me if I did not value you or nurture, or enrich your life in anyway. As I look back on my life except for the first fourteen and the last ten years, I see lives like broken seashells strewn across the seashore of life. Some shattered to small fragments, others with missing pieces but whole, yet other endured the relationship whole on the outside but hurting internally. I pray that you have found the peace and forgiveness necessary to heal, and that mentally, physically and spiritually you are in a good place to help others to come through the vicissitudes of life mentally whole and praising God for: "we know that all things work together for good to them that love God, to them who are the called according to *His* purpose" Rom. 8:28. I apologize and pray and ask for your forgiveness.

To my wife Wilda, who through God's providence has loved me unconditionally, and has supported me through our ups and downs. The journey of life has been greatly enriched by someone who, while they are yet to fully understand me or I her, we have a common belief system and a personal and experiential relationship with God and His son Jesus Christ; which keeps us focused. I have tried several times in the past to build a house based upon my own taste, desire, wants and the world's maxims only to discover that the proverb is true: "Except the LORD build the house, they labour in vain that build it…" Psalms 127:1.

I thank the Lord everyday because not only have I found a wife but in accepting God's choice of a wife for me, I have obtained favor with God. "*Whoso* findeth a wife findeth a good *thing,* and obtaineth favour of the LORD," Prov. 18:22. I know that she is from Him because she is prudent, as His Word has promised: "and a prudent wife *is* from the LORD," Prov. 19:14. With my deepest heartfelt appreciation, love and respect; until death do us part!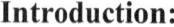

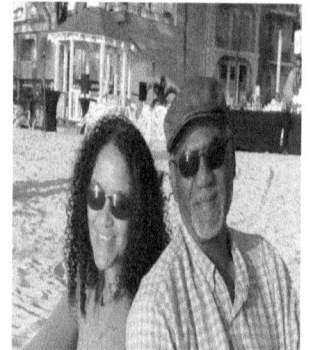

Introduction:

The information presented in this book has been obtained from authentic and reliable sources.

Although great care has been taken to ensure the accuracy of the information presented, the author and the publisher cannot assume responsibility for the validity of all the materials or the consequences of their use. Before starting a regimen of nutritional supplementation, and/or exercise, you should consult a Health Restoration Practitioner proficient in God's Ten Natural Laws of Health.

While it is true that nutrition is the foundation of health, and will again be the leading edge of disease prevention, the information in this book is not intended to tell people to take or stop taking prescription medication. This book is intended to equip the health care consumer with knowledge in conjunction with the advice of a knowledgeable Christian Health Restoration Professional.

It is to this end I pray, that all God fearing peoples but especially Christians will wake up and throw off the cloak of darkness and modern day superstition and trust God with their lives. As Abraham trusted God and was willing to sacrifice Isaac, counting God faithful even unto raising Isaac from the dead. That we will follow God's way of healing even unto the closing of our lives in Christ Jesus and counting God faithful to raise us from the dead at His second coming.

The information in this book is not intended to take the place of competent psychological or psychiatric treatment. It is intended to direct Christians to the correct health care discipline for your health restoration needs. Most of the time the Ten Doctors of nutrition, water, healthy diet, exercise, fresh air, sunshine, temperance, attitude of gratitude, benevolence and trust in God are what a person (true converted Christians) really need. Sometimes the heavy psychotropic Babylonian drugs are necessary (for Babylonians). Sometimes a combination of the two is required, for those with one foot in the church and one foot in the world. Before deciding upon any treatment, medical procedure, or otherwise, obtain two or more professional opinions and then council with God for wisdom.

--Rick L. Lee, N.D, D.D.

God has sent you His Word: "*He sent his word, and healed them (*physically, mentally, spiritually, emotionally, and lifestyle)*, and delivered them from their destructions.*" Based on Psalms 107:20; your only hope as a Christian is in trusting God and following His health plan.

Unintended Consequences:
The statements in this book are not meant to reflect badly on the dedicated staff employed within the sick-care industry, which daily renders compassionate service to the unfortunate sick. The fault and blame clearly lies with John D. Rockefeller, Andrew Carnegie, The American Medical Association, the Pharmaceutical industry and the many governmental agencies and employees of these organizations that turn a blind eye to maintain and up hold a failed system. The Rockefellers', Rothchilds' and Carnegies of the world turned disease into a business, which today we know as the corporate takeover of medicine and incorporated health care as one of the sectors of the U.S. economy, insuring their families' wealth at the expense of the masses. If you would research the American Medical Association (AMA) at the beginning of the 20th century you will find that it was struggling to survive. They organized a council on medical education and tried to make recommendations for improving the professions. By 1908 it had run into committee differences lacking sufficient funds to continue. In 1908 Rockefeller & Carnegie combined efforts & moved with brilliant strategy upon the scene. The president of the Carnegie foundation told the A.M.A. that they would take over and fund the entire project. From the minutes of the A.M.A. council held in N.Y., December of 1908, we find that the Carnegie foundation was too investigate "all the professions; law, [medicine], and theology". According to the report, the profession was to upgrade the inadequacies of medical education. It also made sweeping changes. This gained the A.M.A. tremendous public support. However, two of the suggestions turned out to be unsuspecting hooks. 1. Emphatically strengthen the area of pharmacology and; 2. Bring in additional research departments to all medical schools. That is all medical schools that "qualified". This gave allopathic medicine the advantage over the other health care disciplines because of government funding to those schools that met the requirements. The AMA began to drive out competition. They started by persecuting the Homeopath profession: *"We have never fought the Homeopath on matter of principle. We fought him because he came into our community and got the business."* Dr. J.M. McCormick, AMA, 1903.

As you will learn, this was done out of greed and loyalty to the secret societies they belonged to. There are those also on the European side of the Atlantic like I.G. Farben, Bayer, etc. that are equally responsible, as they all joined together to form the world's biggest cartel. Do not take my word for it, read the following words from a
medical doctor:

"Very few know that the birth hour of the pharmaceutical industry is actually a deliberate decision by a handful of people on this side (Europe) and the other side (America) of the Atlantic Ocean to define disease as a marketplace, and build what has now become the largest investment industry upon that simple thought."

-Dr. Matthias Rath, M.D.

"The thief cometh not, but for to steal, and to kill, and to destroy"... John10:10.

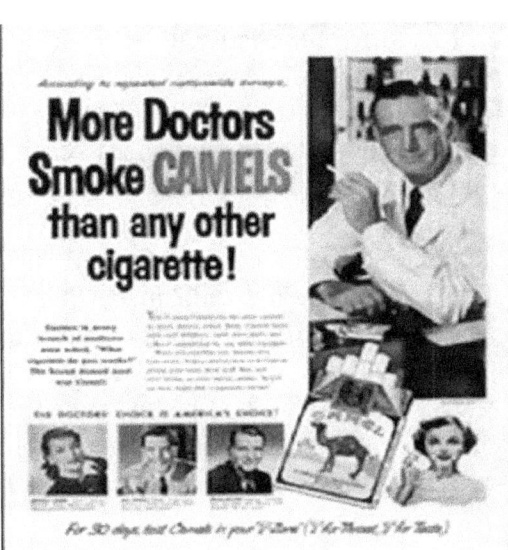

A full page tobacco advertisement like the one to the left was routinely in magazines and periodicals, taken out by the A.M.A, advertised the free use of tobacco as the A.M.A. was heavily funded by the tobacco industry at the time. At the turn of the 19th century the A.M.A. was advertising to the public that tobacco was the answer to all your ills and diseases. The medical profession even prescribed it as a cure for lung disease. It was not until 1957 when a committee of scientists appointed by the American Cancer Society and the American Heart Association conclude that smoking was a causative factor in lung cancer.

Even though many holistic professions like Naturopathy, Homeopathy and others were warning against the use of tobacco. As far back as 1864, nearly 100 years earlier, a Christian health writer wrote: *"Tobacco is a poison of the most deceitful and malignant kind, having an exciting, then paralyzing influence upon the nerves of the body. It is all the more dangerous because its effect upon the system are now slow, and at first scarcely perceivable. Multitudes have fallen victims to its poisonous influence."* Ellen White, Councils on Health, p. 84, 1864. So how do we know that medical science is correct today? It has to be measured against the high standard, of the Word of God! Yes, books like Ministry of Healing, Councils on Diet & Foods, etc…

About the Author

I share the following background information with you to illustrate the severity of mental anguish people experience on a daily basis. As a little boy growing up in Portland Oregon, I was invited into the world of competitive sports by a young pastor names Gerald McCray. Pastor McCray drove through the neighborhood asking young boys if they wanted to play organized basketball, but there was one stipulation, you had to attend the Methodist church he was pastoring in order to play in next week's game. By the time I entered high school, we had already won a city championship.

When I entered high school, I had the opportunity to be a part of, arguably, the best high school men's basketball team in the state of Oregon, as we won two (1971 & 1973) state AAA basketball championships. I was instrumental in helping to win the second championship, being named as a unanimous first team, all tournament selection.

After receiving numerous athletic scholarships from major universities, I chose to stay in state and began my college basketball career. After a successful college career, especially my senior year e.g. being named the most valuable player (MVP) of the 1977 Far West Classic basketball tournament, first team all-Pac 8 1978, being invited to play in the east-west all star game and being selected an honorable mention all-American; I was the third draft selection of the Indiana Pacers, all in 1978.

Personal Experience

Before I can continue, I must interject this about my dad and the reasons why will soon become apparent. Family members and family friends have different perspectives concerning my dad. As an African American male in the tumultuous time that he grew up he remained faithfully married to my mother until the day he died. With the United States government starting its experiment in the African American community called the 'Projects' which was truly an experiment, a project. As welfare check were provided to African American mothers, which encourage them to want the father to leave the home, which bred the absence of the male figure and roll model. I have nothing but respect and admiration for him. My dad was a disciplinarian, principled with honesty and integrity. I know beyond a shadow of a doubt that if it was not for these qualities, I would not be a Christian today.

Now back to my story: My mental and physical anguish began the summer between my freshman and sophomore year of high school, I was fifteen years old. My dad who was not a Christian when I was a little boy became a Christian when I was about ten years old, and joined the Baptist church. It was not until we joined the Seventh-day Adventist church that my world was turned up-side down. That summer the sun shone bright and hot as usual, I went to my favorite parks, swimming at Peninsula Park, went to church and family picnics and attended church on Saturday. At fifteen, with my naive mind, I was not prepared for what was about to befall me and no one prepared me. Fall rolled around and school began, I tried out for football for the first time in my life and became the starting wide-receiver on the junior varsity (J.V.) team. The J.V. team played on Thursdays, so no said a word to me about the Sabbath and not playing sports. Then came November and I was trying out for the men's varsity basketball team, after having a successful freshman season. Like so many young African American males at that time, basketball was my love, and escape. I was already dreaming about playing in the N.B.A. At the time I did not know it but basketball was my god.

    I will never forget it, one Friday evening as the family was preparing for family worship my dad said to me that I could not play basketball on Friday nights. It was the first time in my young life that I questioned my dad. I said what did you say, which was followed by a why. With tears in my eyes, my world came crashing down upon my dreams, hopes and aspirations. My care free easy way of life became frustrating, without realizing it I turned into the typical angry young black male. Basketball kept my out of trouble; my parents always knew where I was, I did not drink alcohol, smoke cigarettes or do drugs. In fact, President Kennedy had started the Presidential Council on Physical Fitness and I had all the posters on my bedroom walls. The theme of the program was "Get High On Sports Not Drugs." My sophomore year in high school I was only able to play J.V. once again, but at the end of the season I was moved up to varsity for the end of the season and the state tournament. At this stage of my life I became introverted; the joking carefree personality was gone and I avoided my dad as much as possible. I was so hurt and angry at him, and with him
working grave yard or swing shift; it was easy for me to not see him
for days at a time until the weekend. The mental and emotional frustration was tremendous, teachers and coaches attempted to talk to my dad with no success. I even called the pastor and asked him if I could keep the Sabbath according to the Hawaiian time zone and was told that was not possible, God expected us to keep the Sabbath according to our location and time. I felt trapped and helpless, my wants, likes, hopes and dreams did not seem to matter. The only thing that seemed to matter was my

blind obedience and loyalty to a religion and God that I did not know or understand and in reality, at the time did not care to know or understand.

My junior year started out the same as the year before by playing J.V. football but when it came time for basketball season; I played on the varsity team. This was a season of lies and deceit with my accomplices being my coaches and family members and family friends. I was not mentally healthy at this stage of my life, wrong became right, self and its desire to play sports became all-absorbing. I played varsity basketball on Friday nights by lying to my dad. I was not the star of the team and drew little attention to myself as far as the sports writers were concerned. My hiding in a sea of high school basketball players all changed my senior year when I blossomed; and my picture began to appear from time to time on the sport page of the newspapers. Letters from universities came to my parents' home offering me a full ride scholarship. Coaches began showing up at my parents' door to discuss my future. It all came crashing down one Friday night when after family worship, I said I was going over to another Seventh-day Adventist friends house for the evening. As my siblings and I were walking out of the living room, my dad without looking up said "boy are you lying to me" and I immediately froze in my tracks as my siblings continued to walk past me.

I replied, very nervously "yes dad I am" I will never forget that Friday night. You see, my father was from a family of eleven siblings and my mother was from a family of nine and no one had ever graduated from college. While my dad kept his emotional composure, I could see the emotional turmoil he was experiencing with the decision before him. We talked, actually he talked and I listened. He did not compromise his position, nor accepted my violating the Sabbath in any way shape or form. After we finished talking, I promptly when up stairs to my bedroom pretending to be going to bed and jumped out of my second story bedroom window and grabbed my duffle bag with my game uniform in it that I had hidden earlier during the day behind a bush next to the house; I walked to the corner where a car was waiting to take me to the gym. The next day my picture was on the sport page of the article written up by the sports writer concerning the game we played Friday night. What happened next totally baffled and bewildered me, I felt totally abandoned and alone. My father came home from work around 10:00 o'clock p.m. to show me the article in the newspaper with my picture then told me that he did not appreciate me lying to him and breaking the rules of his house and ordered me to be out of his house before the next Sabbath. I was confused and stunned, I was not a thief, an addict or even a drug user, and I loved and respected my parents, especially my mother; why was this happening.

The mental stress that I was under today would drive many seventeen year olds to suicide. Later, I found out from one of my siblings that this incident caused a tremendous rift between my parents. Basketball season finally came to an end and I was allowed back into the family home but my relationship my dad would not heal for two and a half decades later.

My senior year finally ended and off to college I went with my anger, bitterness and resentment. These emotions colored my relationships for many decades to come. Failed marriages, tumultuous friendships, fighting on the basketball court during games; and not being free to love because of the anger and distrust that I kept locked in my heart, mind and soul without even realizing that they were there. With my college basketball coming to a close, I was drafted by the Indiana Pacers of the N.B.A. The sun was shining bright as I was on the brink of accomplishing my life time goal and dream, playing in the N.B.A. The roster was trimmed to where one more forward was to be released, the choice came down to Steve Green who played for the University of Indiana or myself. Coach Lenard chose to keep Steve and released me. I remember when I was told the sad news; it was like someone put a dagger into my heart. As I sat in the very last row of seats on the team bus that was taking me to the airport to fly home, with tears running down my face my mind became flooded with the memory of my tumultuous senior year and I broke mentally and physically. I passed through these very dark hours of my life alone, without guidance or support, without a mentor or sibling that had traveled down this path before me. While I thought I was alone and that no one understood, to my family, friends, fans, detractors and myself, it seems as though I had failed. Unbeknown to me at the time, God was working out His master plan in my life.

The next serious mental challenge that took place in my life is when I made the decision to stop playing basketball professionally. I had been playing in Europe under F.I.B.A, the Federation of International Basketball Association. I was home for the summer and staying with my sister and her family, expecting to catch my flight in September back to Europe when my conscience began to bother me. My sister would invite me to church, which I had no interest in but I was driven to research the change of worship from the seventh day of the week, Sabbath to Sunday the first day of the week as Seventh-day Adventist (SDA) claim was done by the Catholic church. So I went to the Multnomah County library in downtown Portland, Oregon. I went up to the fourth or fifth floor to the religious section and began reading the Catholic Encyclopedia and other Catholic books and there it was. Constantine the Emperor of Rome issued the first Sunday Law Decree, which Catholic and most churches today keep in honor of the Catholic Church.

I wished that I had not found the documentation that I was looking for because now, my conscience was really raking me over the coals, I even had trouble sleeping. Then I decided that since the SDA Church has a so called prophet named Ellen White, if I could prove that she was not a prophet then I felt that my conscience would be at peace and I would be free to catch my flight back to Europe. So I began to read and watch everything that I could obtain, both in favor of and against Mrs. White. By the time I concluded my research, I was convicted that she was and is more that a prophet but the messenger of the Lord. I called my agent and told him that I was not going back to Europe and that I was retiring. This was in 1982, ten years removed from my tumultuous senior year in high school when I had rejected Seventh-day Adventism.

That winter in December, I was working a secular job but struggling because that is not what I wanted to be doing, I wanted to be playing basketball and receiving all the perks and amenities that being a sports star brings. I was at the company's Christmas party, the music was playing, food and alcohol was abundant, the people were laughing and really enjoying themselves, all of a sudden I became visibly upset, emotionally. I got a huge lump in my throat and my eyes began to tear up. I immediately left the social and headed for my car. I remember sitting in my car and once again as I did in Indiana losing control of my composure and emotions. As I sat in my car that cold, snowy December night, uncontrollably crying with snot running down my face, I remember telling myself that I was losing my mind. I went into a tale-spin of depression using drugs and alcohol to escape the hurt and pain of reality. I was angry with God, the church, my dad, Coach Lenard and anybody else that I could blame for my failure. Not knowing of mental services and help available through them and probably too proud to used them if I did. My depression deepened, I lost my job, I was acting out, and the anger was ruining relationships. One night while high on marijuana I made a decision that violated my conscience and like the sow when washed goes back to wallow in the mud. I decided to start working out again for another opportunity to try out with a N.B.A. team. The depression immediately left me, I felt hope for the first time in a long time. The picture to the right is Rick at the free throw line in a Clipper's uniform during pre-season. I was excited, focused, and every day I was getting stronger; I got off the drugs (recreational use of marijuana) and alcohol and had a purpose in life again, I thought. My hard work paid off, I was invited to tryout with the then San Diego Clippers of the N.B.A.

Paul Silas was the coach and after a pre-season game against the Denver Nuggets, in which I had to guard all-NBA David Thompson who totally embarrassed me during the game with a monstrous dunk, my adrenaline kicked in and I began to attempt to revenge myself and went against coach Silas' game 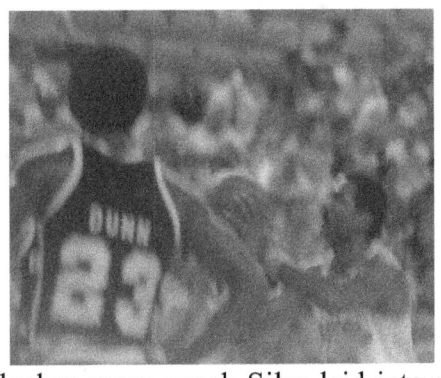 plan. We lost the game and in the locker room coach Silas laid into me and began with verbal expletives. The locker room was so quiet, except for coach Silas' voice that you could hear a pin drop between his breaths. I could not understand why he was so upset at me, we were already down twenty points when he put me into the game, I did not lose the game. Already emotionally charged by the schooling I just received at the hands of Thompson, I felt the anger rise within me and I verbally challenged coach Silas. That was the end of my time with the Clippers. The next day when he called me into his room at the hotel to let me know that he was releasing me, he said that "I could have made the team but that I was a hot head." I apologized and said that a Rickey Lee would never attempt to embarrass a Paul Silas. I turned and walked out the door never again to attempt a N.B.A tryout.

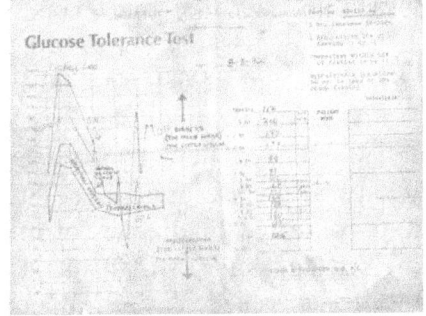

After coming back to Portland and getting a job, it was discovered that I was Diabetic as well. To the left is a picture of my 1982 Glucose Tolerance Test. My blood sugar would go as high as 206 and drop to a low of 38 within a few hours. This test result helped me to understand why at certain times I felt so emotionally out of control and helpless to do anything about it, while the dropping blood sugar issue intensified my irritation problem and the two were a combination for failure. If I was going to make something of myself, be a role model, or mentor then something had to change. One summer, while working as a coach in Darnell Valentine's summer basketball camp at the River Place Athletic Club, in Portland, OR; I was looking at the sea of boys and girls laughing and smiling, enjoying the day, the camp, the friendship of one another; for a moment my mind went back to the days of my youth when everything was so carefree and I enjoyed life. Then my mind went to when everything started getting so very hard and difficult. But before I had the opportunity to wallow in self-pity, my mind went to a statement my grade school basketball coach Phil Walden, who later became a friend, would say to me: "*it is does not matter if you fall, but rather if and how you get up that determines your worth.*" It seemed to me that life had robbed me of my dream, my destiny. I decided right then on that carefree, summer day with the gym full of Children of all sizes and shapes, some awkward, some coordinated and skilled, some overly competitive and other only there for the ice cream; that I was not going to allow life and myself to rob me of my happiness and full potential. I remembered assistant coach Dave Leach in college saying to me that "I was a prima donna." So I began my self assessment by asked my close friends what they thought of me as a person. It was a painful process but I could not cheat or take short cuts. To this day I am very grateful for those who gave me their honest assessment of me.

In a very short time I realized that I had to start at the place it all began, at my rejection of Jesus Christ as my personal savior, and that I had to forgive myself and those who I felt had wronged me, who stole my dream. Now is when I first realized that God was manifesting Himself to me and was helping me to overcome the two greatest challenges of my young life. It was also at this time that I started taking a high quality vitamin and mineral supplement on a daily bases which played a major part in healing my pancreas.

God was working in my life, keeping me from going over the edge. While I was in Europe playing basketball, in a country that I could not speak the language, I had a lot of time to reflect and the Holy Spirit brought me back to my childhood to my dad. I remember everything that he did was for the family. I was six months old when my dad moved to Portland to find work, leaving my mother with four children behind. He could have met another woman and left my mother and us behind, but he was faithful, praise God, reuniting the family at the earliest opportunity. He worked two jobs to support us and was a strong family leader. When he began to question the leaders of the Baptist church as to why they were worshiping on Sunday, I witness the emotional turmoil he experienced as he was asked to leave the church. The Holy Spirit helped me to realize that at every turn, every challenge, and every obstacle he was principled and would not compromise his integrity or violate his conscience. So looking back on my experience at home in high school, I could not have expected him to do anything different than he did, even kicking me out of the family home. I began to write him letters from overseas thanking him for what and who he was and for keeping the family together and apologizing to him for the trouble and pain I caused him. Before he died in 1989 we became closer than we had ever been. I even became closer to him than I was to my mother, who was my support through those difficult years. If my dad had of waivered or compromised, I do not believe that I would be a Protestant, Present Truth, and Seventh-day Adventist today. I am not an SDA because my dad was but because he was my earthly example after he chose to become a Christian and my own research and study of the bible for myself I decided to become a SDA Christian. It has been a struggle and most of it, self inflicted as God has showed me how to *"Let this mind be in you, which was also in Christ Jesus,"* Philippians 2:5.

The key to the Christian struggle is the mind, *"Know ye not, that to whom ye yield yourselves servants to obey, his servants ye are to whom ye obey; whether of sin unto death, or of obedience unto righteousness?"* Romans 6:16.

I quit the team in Europe in December, flew back home no more to play basketball on the Sabbath. This is why SDA who know what they have sacrificed to come into this message cannot tolerate the worldliness and open sins that exist in the church today. We have paid a high price to come into this beautiful Truth and we will remain, by Gods grace loyal to the Truth, not an organization, until the very end.

As one pastor has accurately put it, "the leaders of the organized, corporate church would rather kill the Truth (Jesus) that reform the organization."

Dr. Rick L. Lee, N.D.,
rick@originalhealing.org

The Church of Modern Medicine[1]

"Modern Medicine never calls itself a church. You will never see a medical building dedicated to the religion of medicine; it always says the medical arts, or medical science.

Modern medicine relies on FAITH to survive. All religions do. So heavily does the Church of Modern Medicine rely on FAITH that if everyone somehow simply forgot to believe in it for just one day, the whole system would collapse. For how else could any institution get people to do the things Modern Medicine gets people to do, without introducing a profound suspension of doubt? Would people allow themselves to be artificially put to sleep then cut to pieces in a process they couldn't have the slightest notion about – if they didn't have faith? Would people swallow the thousands of tons of pills a year - again without the slightest knowledge what these chemicals were going to do - if they didn't have faith?

Common to all religions is the claim that reality is not limited to or dependent upon what can be seen, felt, tasted, or smelled. You can easily test modern medical religion on this characteristic by simply asking your doctor WHY enough times. Why are you prescribing this drug? Why is this operation going to do me any good? Why do I have to do that? Why do you have to do that to me?

Just ask WHY and sooner or later you will get to the Chasm of Faith. Your doctor will retreat into the fact that you have no way of knowing or understanding all the wonders he has at his command, and will say "Just Trust Me"!

[1]Confessions of a Medical Heretic, Robert S. Mendelson, M.D. pp, 16, 17.

Chapter I: The Battle Field Is the Mind

The human mind is the battleground for the most deadly conflict ever fought on this planet. Eternal consequences are at stake and we must discern the nature of the battle. The frontal lobe of the brain is the battlefield; whoever controls this part of the brain controls the entire being and their destiny, protect it at all cost!

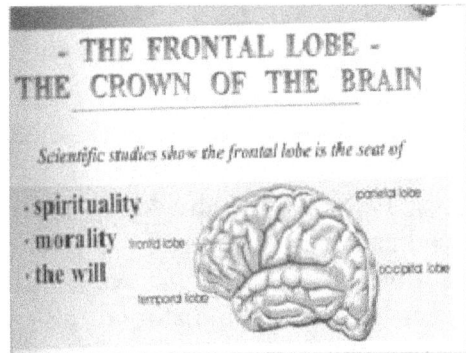

Scientific studies show that the frontal lobe is the crown of the brain. It is the seat of spiritually, *"But the natural man receiveth not the things of the Spirit of God: for they are foolishness unto him: neither can he know them, because they are spiritually discerned."* 1 Cor. 2:14.

It is the seat of your morals, whether right and wrong are fixed laws or is right relative. Are God's Ten Commandment Laws binding upon man or not necessary and placed below man made laws in importance? *"Let us hear the conclusion of the whole matter: Fear God, and keep his commandments: for this is the whole duty of man."* Ecclesiastes 12:13. As well as the strength of our will, not our will power but the will to chose or decide then receive power from God to obey. *"I delight to do thy will, O my God: yea, thy law is within my heart."* Psalms 40:8; and *"Teach me to do thy will; for thou art my God: thy spirit is good; lead me into the land of uprightness."* Psalms 143:10.

The importance of the frontal cannot be emphasized enough as Satan has boasted his capture of it, which means allegiance to him. God has warned us through His word, *"How art thou fallen from heaven, O Lucifer, son of the morning! how art thou cut down to the ground, which didst weaken the nations! For thou hast said in thine heart, I will ascend into heaven, I will exalt my throne above the stars of God: I will sit also upon the mount of the congregation, in the sides of the north: I will ascend above the heights of the clouds; I will be like the most High.* Isaiah 14:12-14. That is Lucifer's, who is now the dragon or Satan's boast. What is most important for you and me, because God will take care of Himself in the conflict against the forces of darkness is that He will protect us as well if we allow Him to. You see Satan boasted that he *"will sit also upon the mount of the congregation, in the sides of the north."*

When you look at the brain the Frontal lobe it is located on the sides of the north. The congregation is God's people and it is Satan's plan to capture, sit (reign), and control your frontal lobe. This why there are so many mental health diseases.

Drugs that Damage our Frontal Lobe
- Illicit drugs
- certain prescription drugs
- other legal social drugs
    - alcohol, nicotine, caffeine,
    - the "ine" cousins, i.e. cocaine, lidocaine, etc.

Drugs that commonly affect the mind: Asthma medications—Beta agonists; blood pressure medication — Beta blockers, calcium channel blockers, centrally acting agents (Clonidine, Methyldopa, etc.); Tranquilizers and sleeping pills—benzodiazepines antidepressants (Note: tricyclic antidepressants are also used for headaches, insomnia, etc.); anti-ulcer pills — H_2-blockers (Tagamet, Zantac); anti-inflammatory drugs — NSAIDS; pain relievers, narcotics; cold and allergy medications — antihistamines (also used for insomnia, etc.), decongestants (especially in children; e.g., pseudoephedrine as in Actifed).

Effects of Compromised Frontal Lobes: Impairment of moral principle, social impairment (loss of love for family), lack of foresight, incapable of abstract reasoning, cannot interpret proverbs, diminished ability for mathematical understanding, loss of empathy, and lack of restraint (boasting, hostility, and aggressiveness).

Frontal Lobe Diseases: Mania, obsessive compulsive disorder, increase appetite, attention deficit/ hyperactivity disorder, and depression. Proof Positive, Neil Nedley, M.D., p. 260.

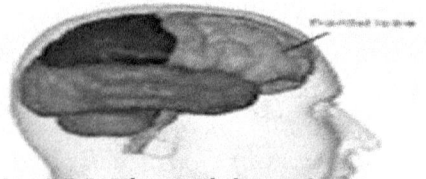
Isa 26:3 Thou wilt keep *him in perfect peace, whose [mind] is stayed on thee: because he trusteth in thee.*

"Thou wilt keep him in perfect peace, whose [mind] is stayed on thee: because he trusteth in thee." Isaiah 26:3.

Mental health includes our emotional, psychological, and social well-being. It affects how we think, feel, and act. It also helps determine how we handle stress, relate to others, and make choices. Mental health is important at every stage of life, from childhood and adolescence through adulthood. Many Factors Contribute to Mental Health Problems:

- Biological factors, such as <u>genes or brain chemistry</u>
- Life experiences, such as trauma or abuse
- Family history of mental health problems

As stated above, genes and brain chemistry play vital roles in mental health problems. One area to consider before giving your love one antipsychotic drugs is Methylenetetrahydrofolate Reductase (MTHFR). MTHFR is due to a genetic mutation that may lead to high levels of homocysteine in the blood and low levels of folate and other vitamins.

Symptoms of a MTHFR mutation
- cardiovascular and thromboembolic diseases (specifically blood clots, stroke, embolism, and heart attacks)
- **depression**.
- **anxiety**.
- **bipolar disorder**.
- **schizophrenia**.
- colon cancer.
- acute leukemia.
- chronic pain and fatigue.

Early Warning Signs of Mental Disease:
- Eating or sleeping too much or too little
- Pulling away from people and usual activities
- Having low or no energy
- Feeling numb or like nothing matters
- Having unexplained aches and pains
- Feeling helpless or hopeless
- Yelling or fighting with family and friends
- Smoking, drinking, or using drugs more than usual
- Feeling unusually confused, forgetful, on edge, angry, upset, worried, or scared
- Experiencing severe mood swings that cause problems in relationships
- Having persistent thoughts and memories you can't get out of your head
- Hearing voices or believing things that are not true
- Thinking of harming yourself or others
- Inability to perform daily tasks like taking care of your kids or getting to work or school.   Mentalhealth.gov.

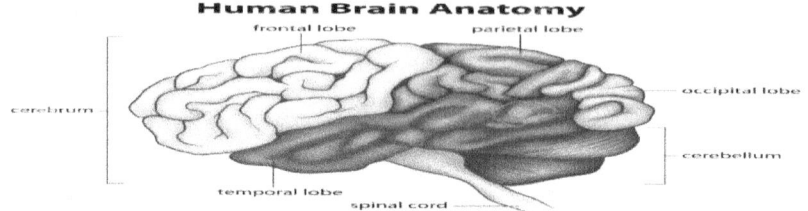

Sickness of the mind prevails everywhere. Nine tenths (9/10) of the diseases from which men suffer have their foundation here.

"Sickness of the mind prevails everywhere. Nine tenths (9/10) of the diseases from which [mankind] suffer from have their foundation here," White, 5T, p. 544.

NEARLY 1 IN 5 AMERICANS SUFFERS FROM MENTAL ILLNESS EACH YEAR, Newsweek BY VICTORIA BEKIEMPIS ON 2/28/14 AT 6:32 PM.

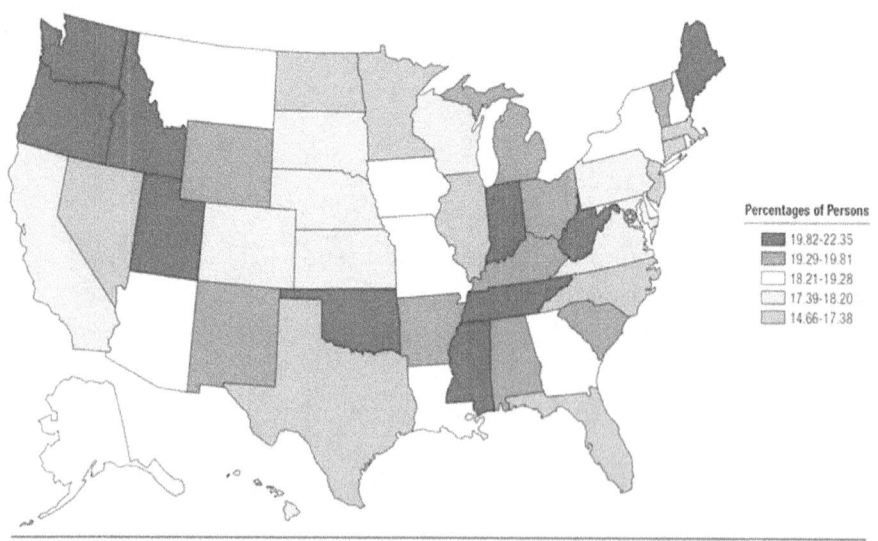

Every year, about 42.5 million American adults (or 18.2 percent of the total adult population in the United States) suffer from some mental illness; enduring conditions such as depression, bipolar disorder or schizophrenia, statistics released Friday reveal. The data, compiled by the Substance Abuse and Mental Health Services Administration (SAMHSA), also indicate that approximately 9.3 million adults, or about

4 percent of those Americans ages 18 and up, experience "serious mental illness" – that is, their condition impedes day-to-day activities, such as going to work.

U.S. Mental Illness Statistics:
- 1 in 4 will experience mental illness
- ½ of the chronic mental illness begin by the age of 14
- ¾ of mental illness begin by the age of 24
- 10.2 million People have co-occurring psychotic disorders along with addictions.
- Depression will be the 2nd leading cause of disability and premature death world wide by 2020
- 1 in 10 Americans take an antidepressant medication

World health report – World Health Organization

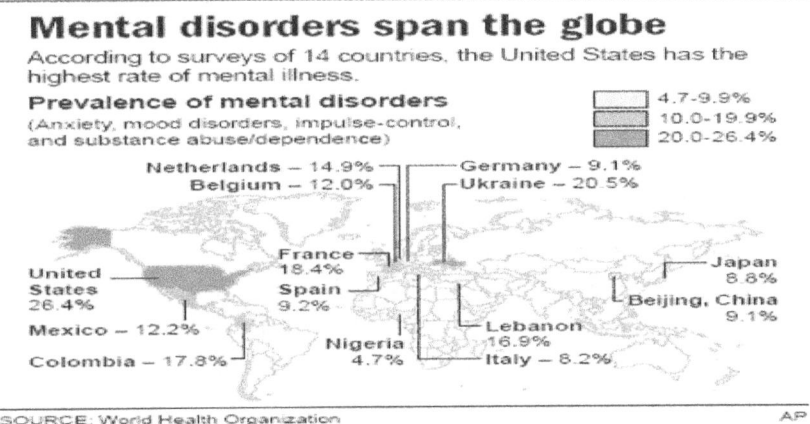

Mental Disorders Affect One in Four People: Geneva, 4 October- One in four people in the world will be affected by mental or neurological disorders at some point in their lives. Around 450 million people currently suffer from such conditions, placing mental disorders among the leading causes of ill-health and disability worldwide.

The conflict is raging, minds are being captured and destroyed, fulfilling the prophecy of Revelation 18:23, "…for by thy sorceries were all nations deceived. The stress of society with its attempted escape through recreational and medical marijuana, marital, educational and family dysfunction is putting undue pressure on individual minds. Nations are very angry causing an intensity of uncertainty unparalleled in human history, causing men, women and children hearts/minds to fail; *"Men's hearts failing them for fear, and for looking after those things* which are coming on the earth: for the powers of heaven shall be shaken," Luke 21:26.

God has created the body for the purpose of the mind; to weaken the former destroys the latter. "*God has prepared this living habitation for the mind. It is curiously wrought, a temple which the Lord himself has fitted up for the indwelling of the Holy Spirit. The mind controls the whole man. All our actions, good or bad, have their source in the mind. It is the mind that worships God, and allies us to heavenly beings. All the physical organs are the servants of the mind, and the nerves are the messengers that transmit its orders to every part of the body, guiding the motions of the living machinery.*" White, FE, p. 403.4

The enemy of your mental and physical health knows and understands God's health principles better than we. The book 'No Healing Medicines' reveals Satan's attack on the physical to gain control of the mental, in order to destroy the spiritual. The adversary knows that if he can weaken the body or physical power he will be successful in the overthrow of your faith. "*The body is the only medium through which the mind and the soul are developed for the up building of character. Hence it is that the adversary of souls directs his temptations to the enfeebling and degrading of the physical powers. His success here means the surrender to evil of the whole being. The tendencies of our physical nature, unless under the dominion of a higher power, will surely work ruin and death*," White, CDF, p. 73.

Chapter II: His Servant ye are to whom ye obey

The human mind is the battleground for the deadliest conflict ever fought on this planet. Satan is playing the game of life for the souls of men. "There are but <u>two powers that control the minds of men</u>-- the power of God and the power of Satan," Temperance, p. 276. Let us attempt to analyze how the two great powers of good and evil work.

1) Christ seeks to control our minds so that we might reach the highest fulfillment of the capabilities that He, Himself, built into that marvelous organ.
2) Satan, on the other hand, seeks to retain control of that mind which is "enmity against God." Romans 8:7.
3) "Because the carnal mind *is* [enmity] against God: for it is not subject to the law of God, neither indeed can be," Romans 8:7. G2189 Strong's Hebrew & Greek Dictionaries, ἔχθρα, echthra, ekh'-thrah
   Feminine of <u>G2190</u>; *hostility*; by implication a reason for *opposition:* - <u>enmity, hatred</u>.
4) "*Christ is the source of every right impulse*," SC, p. 26.

5) "<u>Satan is ever seeking to impress and control the mind</u>, and none of us are safe except as we have a constant connection with God," 4T. p. 542.1.
6) "*Satan takes control of every mind that is not decidedly under the control of the Spirit of God*," TM, p. 79.

King Solomon – Socrates

"For as he thinketh in his heart, so *is he*..."
-- King Solomon, Psalms 27:3.

"As a man thinketh, so is he." — **Socrates**

Socrates was echoing King Solomon words recorded in the Bible seven hundred years earlier.

Thinking has such a profound in pack on our lives that we really need to guard the avenues to our souls. *"Those who would not fall a prey to Satan's devices, must guard well the avenues of the soul; they must avoid reading, seeing, or hearing that which will suggest impure thoughts. The mind must not be left to dwell at random upon every subject that the enemy of souls may suggest. The heart must be faithfully sentineled, or evils without will awaken evils within, and the soul will wander in darkness."* White, CDF, p. 73.

Our thinking can even modify our genes.
--John Eccles, Neuroscientist, Clinical & Experimental Hypertension; Theory & Practice, 6, 63-78, 1984.

"For as he thinketh in his heart, so *is he*" take on new and profound meaning with such research!

God's Plan
Come now, and let us reason together, saith the LORD... Isa. 1:18, is the basis of God's plan for working with the human family. *"God first requires the heart, the affections."* 2T, p. 169. (The mind and the heart are used interchangeably in Scripture as well as in the Spirit of Prophecy). An example of this is "For as he thinketh in his heart, so *is he*... Prov. 23:7. Often it is said about someone who is learning how to become a Christian, "All that he has left to do is give up this or that bad habit." Possessions, attitudes or habits of life do not constitute the problem; they are only symptoms of the real problem. God says"... man looketh on the outward appearance, but the Lord looketh on the heart." 1 Samuel 16:7. Keep thy heart with all diligence; for out of it *are* the issues of life, Prov. 4:23.

"As the leaven, when mingled with the meal, works from within outward, so it is by the renewing of the heart that the grace of God works to transform the life. No mere external change is sufficient to bring us into harmony with God. There are in many who try to reform by correcting this or that bad habit, and they hope in this way to become Christians, but they are beginning in the wrong place. "<u>Our first work is with the heart</u>." COL. p. 97.1, Also see 1SM. p. 353.

The decision we must make is to allow the mind of Christ to become ours. "Let this mind be in you, which was also in Christ Jesus," Philp. 2:5. We must make this decision because "…you, that were sometime alienated and <u>enemies in *your* mind by wicked works</u>, yet now hath he [reconciled]" Colossians 1:21.

We can readily see that God's method of accomplishing His goal for man is to begin with the heart/mind. Even this must be by our willing permission. Behold, I stand at the door, and knock: if any man hear my voice, and open the door, I will come in to him… Rev. 3:20.

"If ye be willing and obedient, ye shall eat the good of the land." Isaiah 1:19.

"… *God will accept only willing service*, SDABC, vol. 7, p. 977. Therefore, He cannot accept obedience that is the result of obligation, force, or even the desire to satisfy a guilty conscience.

"The man who attempts to keep the commandments of God from a sense of obligation merely--because he is required to do so--will never enter into the joy of obedience. He does not obey. When the requirements of God are accounted a burden because they cut across human inclination, we may know that the life is not a Christian life. True obedience is the outworking of a principle within. It springs from the <u>love of righteousness, the love of the law of God</u>. The essence of all righteousness is loyalty to our Redeemer. This will lead us to do right because it is right--because right doing is pleasing to God". COL 97.3.

Satan's Methods

Satan's method of working began in heaven where he was successful in his efforts to spread the rebellion that began in his own mind: "*It was his policy to perplex with subtle arguments concerning the purposes of God. Everything that was simple he shrouded mystery, and by artful perversion cast doubt upon the plainest statements of Jehovah,*" PP. p. 41.

His plan has worked so well that he has carried it out here on earth for nearly six thousand years.

"The enemy is a master worker, and if God's people are not constantly led by the Spirit of God, they will be snared and taken. For

thousands of years Satan has been experimenting upon the properties of the human mind, and he has learned to know it well. By his subtle workings in these last days, he is linking the human mind with his own, imbuing it with his thoughts; and he is doing this work in so deceptive a manner that those who accept his guidance know not that they are being led by him at his will. The great deceiver hopes to so confuse the minds of men and women, that none but his voice will be heard," 2SM. p. 352, 353.

"Satan's work began in heaven by suggesting doubts, questions and thoughts in such a subtle way that the unfallen angels were not aware that they were being led by Him. They uttered thoughts that originated with him, thinking they were their own," PP, p. 35-40.

Any plan that worked so well in heaven would surely work well on earth. We are witnesses to its success. Now let us analyze these plans together. Both powers are seeking complete control of the mind to the exclusion of the other; God, by man's willing surrender to Him, Satan by man's insistence on independence—a gift from the devil himself.

"The enemy is preparing for his last campaign against the church. He has so concealed himself from view that many can hardly believe that he exists, much less can they be convinced of his amazing activity and power. They have to a great extent forgotten his past record; and when he makes another advance move, they will not recognize him as their enemy, that old serpent, but they will consider him a friend, one who is doing a good work. Boasting of their independence they will, under his specious, bewitching influence, obey the worst impulses of the human heart and yet believe that God is leading them. Could their eyes be opened to distinguish their captain, they would see that they are not serving God, but the enemy of all righteousness. <u>They would see that their boasted independence is one of the heaviest fetters Satan can rivet on unbalanced minds</u>," 5T. p. 294.1.

If the Son therefore shall make you free, ye shall be free indeed, John 8:36.

At the very highest level within the mind of man God placed His most precious gift—the will.

"This is the governing power in the nature of man, the power of decision, or of choice. Everything depends on the right action of the will", SC, p. 47.

"Your will is the spring of all your actions", MYP, p. 135, 5T, p. 513-516.

With such a power in Satan's control how easy it would be to bring man to destruction, while deceiving him into thinking he could change as he desired.

> "<u>This will, that forms so important a factor in the character of man, was at the fall given into the control of Satan</u>; and he has ever since been working in man to will and to do of his own pleasure, but to the utter ruin and misery of man". 5T, p. 513-516.

This is the exact the same method he used in heaven. Here is Satan's control without his involvement even being recognized. Satan knows that God will not remove this control from him, for God will never force our will. Because of God's gift of giving Jesus Christ to mankind as part of the plan of salvation, God can say, "*Yield yourself up to Me; give Me that will; take it from the control of Satan, and I will take possession of it; then I can work in you to will and to do of My good pleasure.*" MYP, p. 154, 5T, p. 513-516.

In order to stop sinning, ("Whosoever is born of God doth not commit sin; for his seed remained in him: and he cannot sin, because he is born of God." 1 John 3:9), we must take our will back from Satan and give it to God. Satan well knows that he cannot retain or force man's will if man chooses to remove it from his control.

> "*The tempter has no power to control the will or to force the soul to sin,*" GC. p, 510.

As long as Christ is in control, Satan is powerless.
> "*Satan knows that he cannot overcome man unless he can control the will,*" Te, p. 16.

> "*The tempter can never compel us to do evil. He cannot control minds unless they are yielded to his control. The will must consent, faith must let go its hold upon Christ, before Satan can exercise his power upon us,*" DA, p. 125.2.

Here lies Satan's weakness!
> "*Satan is well aware that the weakest soul who [abides] in Christ is more than a match for the hosts of darkness, and that, should he reveal himself openly, he would be met and resisted,*" GC. p, 530.

When struggling with addiction(s) the mind must remember and believe God promises. "But as many as received him, to them gave He power to become the sons of God, *even* to them that believe on his name" John 1:12, etc...

It must be understood that while we can remove our will from Satan, we have no power to keep it ourselves. It must be surrendered completely to Jesus, or Satan will take control again.

"No man can serve two masters: for either he will hate the one, and love the other; or else he will hold to the one, and despise the other. Ye cannot serve God and mammon," Matt. 6:24.

"None but Christ can fashion anew the character that has been ruined by sin. He came to expel the demons that had controlled the will," DA. p. 38.

We must understand how Satan and his evil angels gain access to our will in order to control it.

"<u>Those who would not fall a prey to Satan's devices, must guard well the avenues of the soul; they must avoid reading, seeing, or hearing that which will suggest impure thoughts</u>. The mind must not be left to dwell at random upon every subject that the enemy of souls may suggest. The heart must be faithfully sentineled, or <u>evils without will awaken evils within</u>, and the soul-mind will wander in darkness," AA. p. 518.

"All should guard the senses, lest Satan gain victory over them; for these are the avenues of the soul-mind," AH, p. 401.

"It is <u>through the will that sin retains its hold upon us</u>. The surrender of the will is represented as plucking out the eye or cutting off the hand, TMB, p. 61.

"And if thy right hand offend thee, cut it off, and cast *it* from thee: for it is profitable for thee that one of thy members should perish, and not *that* thy whole body should be cast into hell," Matt. 5:30.

If you have never thought to take your will from Satan's control, why not do it right now? Just say audibly to Satan, "I am taking my will from your control and surrendering it to Jesus." Then say to Jesus, "Please take my will for I cannot keep it." Then work in accordance with your prayer. *"Let everyone show his faith by his works."Faith without works is dead," "being alone."* RH, Aug. 8. 1894

"*When you give up your own will, your own wisdom, and learn of Christ, you will find admittance into the kingdom of God*," 1SM, p. 110.

There is no power in heaven or hell that can force us to take this simple step. However, if you do not, you are under the control of Satan, even though you do not see him and you boast of your independence. Once you have surrendered to Christ, then you have to daily abide in Him, John 15:4.

How we abide in Christ:
"*I am the vine, ye are the branches. Can we conceive of a more intimate relation to Christ than this? The fibers of the branch are almost identical with those of the vine. The communication of life, strength, and fruitfulness from the trunk to the branches is unobstructed and constant. The root sends its nourishment through the branch. Such is the true believer's relation to Christ. He abides in Christ, and draws his nourishment from Him.*" ML, p. 11.2.

"*This spiritual relation can be established only by the exercise of personal faith. This faith must express on our part supreme preference, perfect reliance and entire consecration. Our will must be wholly yielded to the divine will; our feelings, desires, interests, and honor, identified with the prosperity of Christ's kingdom and the honor of His cause, be constantly receiving grace from Him, and Christ accepting gratitude from us.*" ML, p. 11.3.

Chapter III: Psychiatry: God's blessing or Man's Curse
Insurance companies pay out sixty nine billion dollars a year in insurance premiums for psychiatric services, doubling the cost of medical insurance premiums. While raking in over 2 trillion annually, psychiatrist cannot point to a single cure. Hard to believe, that is exactly what they count on; this how psychiatry and medicine as a whole has been getting away with it from the very beginning.

"*The roots of psychiatry have to do with control, power and alienation from certain groups of people who are uncomfortable to be around; they were locked up in these places to get them out of the way*".
--Dr. Lee Coleman, Author – Reign of Error.
Psychiatry has gotten into every facet of our lives. "*The Psychiatry industry believes that everyone is mentally ill*". –Dr. Jeffery Schaler, Professor, Dept. of Justice & Law; American University.

"If you smoke to much it is a disease, if you are too happy it is a disease, if you are too thin it is a disease, if you are too fat it is a disease".—Dr. Thomas Szasa, Professor and Author "The Myth of Mental Illness".

"Were are these things coming from? They are coming from the minds of psychiatrist who are dreaming them up. Writing papers and getting them published and getting their names on it, creating these new diseases". – Dr. Mark Filidei, Director Medical Clinic

"There is not one shred of creditable evidence that any respectable scientist would consider valid demonstrating that anything that psychiatrist call mental diseases, brain diseases, or chemical imbalances, it's all fraud". –Dr. Ron Leifel, Psychiatrist.

"There is no liability of diagnoses and there is science, just pseudo-science, it is pretend science".—Dr. Margaret Hagen, Prof. of Psychology, Boston University.

"This is one of the most open secrets in all of America in the psychiatric field, that nothing, nothing that is being done is legitimate and they are billing for it".—Gary Null, Prof. of Science, Fairleigh Dickerson University.

Psychiatrists claim that over one billion of the world's population is mentally ill. In the Past thirty five years the number of people taking psychiatric drugs has tripled to over 120 million users today (2006). Right now, they drug 20 million school children with stimulants and other psychotropic drugs.

At a recent American Psychiatric Association convention when asked about the scientific bases of their profession, those psychiatrics who would be interviewed offered nothing but excuses.
        –Citizens Commission on Human Rights

"Psychiatric illness is not really an illness". –Psychiatrist Germany

"How do you evaluate if someone is cured or sick"?
                                        --Psychiatrist Mexico

"A cure is certainly something we look forward to and we have no earthly idea how to accomplish".   Psychiatrist United States

"We are not good at causes; we don't know what causes mental illness".
– Psychiatrist Norway

But that has not stopped them from calling themselves mental health experts and treating people against their will.
–Citizens Commission on Human Rights.

"It is really tragic, it's awful and it is being done for money that is why it is being done". --Robert Whitaker, Author, Mad In America.

"Oh it is big, so big, I don't know the exact figures but it's huge". Kelly O'Meara, Journalist and Author.

"This is so big that it boggles the mind".
Dr. Thomas Szasa, Professor and Author "The Myth of Mental llness".

Since 1965 nearly twice as many Americans died in government psychiatric hospitals than U.S. soldiers killed in battle, in all wars since 1775 to 2010, over 1.1 million psychiatric deaths. The U.S. government and private insurers' payout one hundred billion dollars every year for psychiatric services, substantially inflating the cost of medical insurance

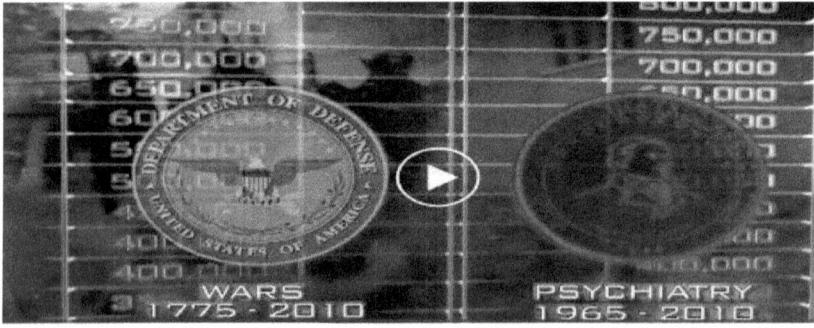

premiums, while raking in a third of a trillion dollars ($6,792,034,958.00) annually, psychiatry cannot point to a single cure. Hard to believe, that is exactly what they count on. That is how they have been getting away with it from the very beginning.
–Citizens Commission on Human Rights (cchr.org).

Diagnostic & Statistical Manuel of Mental Disorders (DSM)

In the early 1950's Diagnostic & Statistical Manuel of Mental Disorders was compiled, largely from the work of a German by the name of Emil Kreapelin, Psychiatrist from the 1890's; who was first credited with classification of mental disorders. He was the first person to classify what he thought were biological classifications of the brain. An interesting fact is that he only identified three mental disorders, Dementia Praecox, which is now called schizophrenia; Manic-depressive illness and Paranoid Psychosis. All of which are concepts that still exist in the DSM today, yes only three.

"The DSM uses very little statistics in the book and disorder is used essentially as a euphuism for illness. This is a book that catalogs mental illnesses for which no medical sign has ever been discovered".
--Robert Spillane, Professor of Psychology

According to psychiatrist, any part of life can be labeled a mental disorder. This comes right out of the Diagnostic & Statistical Manuel of Mental Disorders; it is 943 pages and list out 374 mental "disorders". It lists everything from depression and anxiety to stuttering, cigarette addiction, fear of spiders, nightmare disorder, math disorder, and even a disorder of infancy. All reinterpreted and many ,
falsely labeled as a brain disease. It is the basis for the listing of mental disorders in the International Classification of Diseases that is used throughout the world. And though it weighs less than five pounds, its influence pervades all aspects of modern society: our governments, our courts, our military, our media and our schools. Using it, psychiatrists can enforce psychiatric drugging, seize your children and even take away your most precious personal freedoms. It is psychiatry's Diagnostic and Statistical Manual of Mental Disorders, and it is the engine that drives a $330 billion psychiatric industry.

But is there any proof behind the DSM? Or is it nothing more than an elaborate pseudoscientific sham? --Citizens Commission on Human Rights (cchr.org).

Yes people have problems but psychiatrists reduce everything down to something wrong with the brain. Psychiatrists have a book of life's problems reinterpreted as mental disorders, which is not based or backed by science. At the 163rd annual American Psychiatric Association convention this startling revelation was made: *"The DSM is made up of committees of men who have political opinions and women who have biases and political opinions, so there is not nearly as much science in DSM as there should to be"*. Psychiatrist, North Dakota.

"Like at the previous (DSM) meeting people met in the bathroom and decided that something should be in there and then they would go and propose it to the whole committee". --Psychiatrist, Resident Texas.

"You have this kind of lumping of several observations and when you get enough of them in one tent, you've got a diagnosis. --Psychiatrist, Iowa.

"*The DSM system is not the real system of diagnoses*", --Psychiatrist, Sweden.

"*A lot of the diagnoses in there have not been rigorously validated*".
--Psychiatrist, Resident Texas.

"It is the best tool that we have available but it is not perfect".
--Psychiatrist, District of Columbia.

"*It is so useless that if you give me a patient and the DSM, I'll make at least 20 diagnoses on the same patient*". --Psychiatrist, Illinois.

"*You have to take it with a grain of salt*". --Psychiatrist, Pennsylvania.

"*It is actually getting more and more complicated*". --Psychiatrist, England.

"**We are left with diagnosing things based upon check lists and questionnaires, which sort of leaves us out of the rest of medicine because we do not have a biological test**." Psychiatrist, Massachusetts.

The lack of science in the DSM is actually an open secret; here is what some professionals have to say about it.

"*The DSM is actually a scam; it has been described as a house of cards. Why? Because the diagnose are theoretical, they are not based on scientific measurements*". --Dr. Anna Law, Emergency Room Physician.

"*The DSM is sort of a shaky level built upon another shaky level, built upon another shaky level*". --Thomas Glick, Attorney.

"*The DSM is flimsy, easily collapsible under the scrutiny of critical thinking*" --Robert Spillane, Professor of Psychology.

"*If you just pull one little fragment of the reasoning aside and questioning thoroughly and you will find that it does not stand up then that means that the whole organism collapse because you got some wrong premise in *there somewhere. In fact they are all over the place".* --Dr. Peter Mansfield, Physician.

"It is indeed a house of cards because it is not predicated on a solid structure. It is built to appear as a legitimate edifice, but any serious inquiry will show it to be illegitimate. --Jonathan Emord, Attorney

Diagnostic & Statistical Manuel of Mental Disorders II (DMS-II) came along in 1968 and expanded to 178 disorders, which gained for them even more government insurance funding. To gain international recognition MDS-II was specifically written to align with the International Statistic Classification of Disease and other Health Problems (ICD), today ICD-10. A book used extensively in Europe and around the world that apart from Psychiatric disorders, list real medical diseases. So that is how psychiatric disorders got accepted in mainstream medicine. It was a start but the DMS-II was still not scientific as it was heavenly influenced but not by clinical testing but by the theories of Austrian psychologist Sigmund Freud. Then there must have been a lot of neuroses, yep but there was absolutely no knowledge of what caused them, nor did they even look for a cause.

"Inclusion of a disorder in the Classification "does *not require* that there be knowledge about its etiology [cause]." In other words to make a diagnoses you really do not need to bother with cause and effect. You do not need to know what causes the condition. --Bret Hartman, Clinical Psychologist.

If the DSM does not tell you the cause of a mental disorder then how do psychiatrists discover them in the first place? The answer may surprise you.

"New diseases are being invented all the time and I want to emphasize the word, invented. Because when it comes to Psychiatry mental illnesses are not discovered there invented". --Jeffrey Schaler, Professor of Psychology American University.

How the system works in terms of diagnoses it that, every few years a group of psychiatrist and psychologist sit around in a room and vote on new diagnoses. --Craig Newnes, Clinical Psychologist.

There is more, not only are mental disorders voted into the DSM, but now and then they are voted out. Take for example h homosexuality, listed in DMS one and two as a mental illness. This is how the editor and chief of DSM-III explains it.

"I came up with a definition in 1973 [that made it possible to argue] that homosexuality was not a mental disorder". Dr. Robert Spitzer, Editor in Chief, DSM-III.

"On a vote essentially at a conference of the American Psychiatric Association, homosexuality was removed." Robert Spillane, Professor of Psychology.

"Now did they discover that homosexuality was not a disease through scientific processes, no, it was included for political reasons and it was removed for political reasons".--Jeffrey Schaler, Professor of Psychology, American University.

"It is done as a supposed democracy, so to call it science is a complete fabrication". --Brent Hartman, Clinical Psychologist.

The DSM is political and not scientific, right!!!

Shuffling the Deck – Repackaging the DSM

Psychiatry wanted to be seen as doctors they still were not accepted into mainstream medicine, so that is why they decided the next edition would look much more scientific. They decided the DSM's next edition was going to be completely different. It was a decision that would change psychiatry forever.

"If you roll the clock forward to the 1970's in the United States, at that time psychiatry was in very poor shape, for a number of reasons. First of all it was held in very low regard by other members of the medical profession, so psychiatry was something you did if you could not succeed in any other area of medicine; and people such as Robert Spitzer, Editor in Chief, DSM-III in America made it very clear that the time had come essentially that psychiatrist of medicine should practice medicine". –Richard Benthall, Professor of Clinical Psychology.

Diagnostic & Statistical Manuel of Mental Disorders III (DMS-III)

"So if psychiatrist were spending a lot of time with people, say who were anxious, depressed, these dilemmas, these problems in living essentially had to be redefined and they were redefined as medical conditions". --Robert Spillane, Professor of Psychology.

"Their solution for this was to come up with a manual to Psychiatric disorders more carefully. So hence, we have DSM-III, which is the third edition and was published in 1980". –Richard Benthall, Professor of Clinical Psychology.

Under Robert Spitzer, Psychiatrist editing the DSM-III throughout Freudian psychology and agreed that from now on psychiatrist diagnoses were purely biological. So they finally became scientific, No, actually not at all, in fact the political bickering over what disorders to put in and what to leave out of the DSM-III was even more ridiculous. Here is what one psychiatrist had to say about it:

"They would squeeze into a room which was about half the size of this one. It was much too small and Bob (Robert Spitzer) would raise a provocative question and people would shout out their opinions from all sides of the room. Whoever shouted the loudest tended to be heard. My own impression is it was more like a tobacco auction than a sort of conference. –Dr. David Shaffer, Psychiatrist.

This is what another member of the DSM decision making panel said "The low level of intellectual effort was shocking. Diagnoses were developed by the majority vote on the level we would use to choose a restaurant. You feel like Italian, I feel like Chinese, so let's go to a cafeteria. Then it's typed into the computer. It may reflect on our naiveté, but it was our belief that there would be an attempt to look at things scientifically." —Renee Carfinkel, Psychologist.

It looks like they had a manual that looked scientific but was no more scientific than before. Mean while, the number of mental disorders had ballooned to 259, but to sell the idea that Psychiatry was a true medical science they had to spin it with a really impressive scientific sounding theory.

"But with DSM-III from 1980 on, it was the progressive medicalization of psychiatry. The notion of chemical imbalance was invented and eventually took hold". -- Robert Spillane, Professor of Psychology.

Is there such a thing as a chemical imbalance in the brain that can cause psychological problems?

"No, actually that is one of the misstatements of disinformation, or misinformation that is coming out and unfortunately, I think a psychologist believes that there is a chemical imbalance and a lot of people do. Psychologist, educators, the psychiatrics certainly accept it, now pediatrician are accepting it. It is not caused by a chemical imbalance and what makes me the angriest is that so many of the doctors are just buying in to that. It's just not true".

-David B. Steib, Ph.D., Clinical Psychologist.

Is there a test that can be performed to determine if there is a chemical imbalance?

"They claim that they have found this chemical imbalance or that anatomical problem, or anomaly with the brain or nervous system and yet if you were to send your child to a lab to have the chemical test done on his blood or urine, they would look at you like you are insane because it cannot be done. So what they claim as an imbalance cannot be measured by any laboratory urine test or Positron emission tomography (PET) scans, or computed tomography (CT or CAT) scan; none of it can be replicated at the clinical level. There are about a thousand claims that come out every year, where they think that they have found the cause of depression, or ADD, or bipolar disorder, none of it is true. --David B. Steib, Ph.D., Clinical Psychologist.

"As a parent you search for honest answers, and if you go to the book store the books would say the same thing, the same garbage would be inundated in the book shelves and you pull book after book and they all say the same thing, chemical imbalance, neurological disorder and they need the drugs and the therapies combinations is the way to go. You would have gotten it from everywhere you would have looked except the very few scholars around the nation and the world that are fighting this and we are a rare breed. We read deep into literature, as a parent you are not at fault for what happened or happens to your child if you do not know this information. Now the prevailing and pervasive attitude is what society walks into. --David B. Steib, Ph.D., Clinical Psychologist. For more information go to cchr.com.

Psychiatry and Psychology like modern medicine is built upon a false theory for the financial benefit of the few at the expense of yours and my love ones. Nutrition and God's ten doctors are the best answer for anyone road to recovery.

Poor Mental Health, a Nutritional Deficiency?
God's remedies are the simple agencies of nature that will not tax or debilitate the system through their powerful properties. Pure air and water, cleanliness, a proper diet, purity of life, and a firm trust in God are remedies for the want of which thousands are dying; yet these remedies are going out of date because their skillful use requires work that the people do not appreciate. Fresh air, exercise, pure water, and clean, sweet premises are within the reach of all with but little expense, 5T p. 443.1.

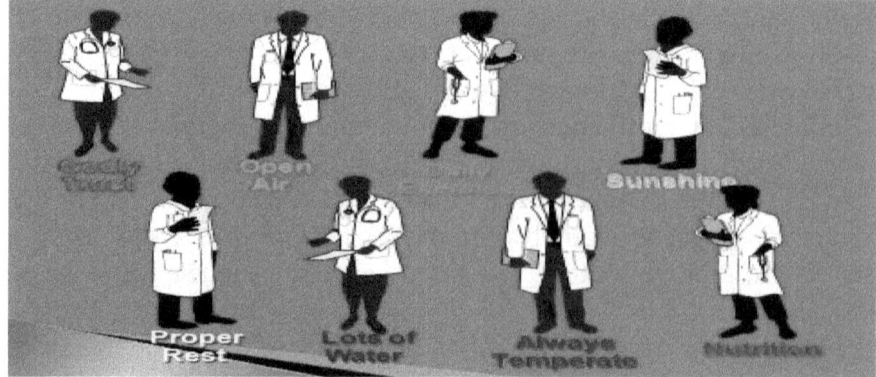

"Who forgiveth all thine iniquities; who healeth all thy diseases" Psalms 103:3.

Dr. Nutrition

It is a fact 99% of all Americans are deficient in organic minerals because "inorganic (i.e., toxic, synthetic, dead, and inert) Chemicals, pesticides, and herbicides have destroyed nearly all the critical organic complexes, elements and minerals in our soil.

1. The nutritional and food industries knew that nutritional deficient food was coming to us from the farm lands (1936).
2. They realized that processing was further robbing us of trace minerals that could be found (1940's).
3. They knew we were cooking any remaining nutrients right out of our food.

When you heat or cook food you start to kill the micro nutrients at 112° F, at 118° F you start to kill off enzymes.

In other words, the U.S. government has known for over 70 years that nutrient depleted food was coming to the tables of U.S. families. *74th Congress: Finding Presented in U.S. Senate Document 264, written and published in 1936.*

Two time Nobel Prize winner Linus Pauling made this statement: *"Every element, every sickness, and every disease can be traced back to an organic trace mineral deficiency."* –Linus Pauling (categorical statement).

Matthew 19:6 tells us, "What therefore God hath joined together, let not man put asunder." What therefore includes grains and/or foods. Now, a grain of wheat has over twenty two different nutrients in it, if left alone. The United States (U.S.) government has known since 1936 that low and/or nutritionally depleted soil was producing nutritionally depleted food. Now enters upon the scene modern food processing which began in the 1940, to extend the shelf life of food products. Food processors seem more interested in shelf life than human life. By removing the bran and germ of wheat, flour can be made into bread that won't spoil as quickly. This process, however, removes 22 vitamins and other nutrients. Soon scientists discovered that this processed flour was causing B1, B2, B3 and iron deficiencies in the American population. Therefore, Congress passed the Enrichment Act of 1948 that forced food processors to add these four nutrients back into the flour they "refined."

Today the majority of food manufactures use a synthetic form of iron in their food products.

Eating Poorly a Factor in 1 in Every 5 Deaths Worldwide

"Diet is a factor in one of every five deaths around the world. That means millions of people are consuming too much salt and sugar and not enough whole grains, fruits, seeds, nuts and vegetables."

--The *Global Burden of Disease* study

Can what you eat affect your mental health? New research links diet and the mind. By Gisela Telis March 24, 2014

Jodi Corbitt had been battling depression for decades and by 2010 had resigned herself to taking antidepressant medication for the rest of her life. Then she decided to start a dietary experiment. To lose weight, the 47-year-old Catonsville, Md., mother stopped eating gluten, a protein found in wheat and related grains. Within a month she had shed several pounds — and her lifelong depression.

"It was like a veil lifted and I could see life more clearly," she recalled. "It changed everything." Corbitt had stumbled into an area that scientists have recently begun to investigate: whether food can have as powerful an impact on the mind as it does on the body. Research exploring the link between diet and mental health "is a very new field; the first papers only came out a few years ago," said Michael Berk, a professor of psychiatry at the Deakin University School of Medicine in Australia. "But the results are unusually consistent, and they show a link between diet quality and mental health."

The Washington Post, Health & Science, May 24, 2014

For the complete and very interesting article google or bing: washingtonpost.com/national/health-science/can-what-you-eat-affect-your-mental-health.

"The human body heals itself and nutrition provides the resources to accomplish the task." – Roger Williams

How to heal the broken brain with Dr. Nutrition and Natures other natural doctors.

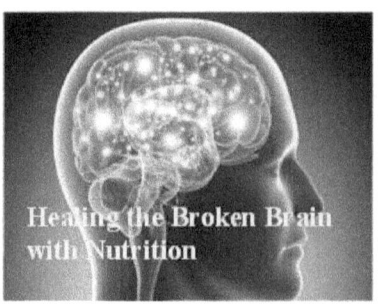
Healing the Broken Brain with Nutrition

A healthy brain requires eleven different minerals to function properly: Calcium, Magnesium, Iodine, Iron, Manganese, Phosphorus, Potassium, Flourine, Silicon, Sulphur and Zinc = 11. This does not include enzymes, antioxidants, flavonoids and bioflavonoids, etc... The most alarming fact not readily known, shared or understood by the majority of people, is the human body cannot make its own minerals. We are completely dependent on outside sources for our mineral nutrition. From the day we are born, our mineral stores begin to deplete and if we are not replenishing them with what we put into our bodies, in the correct form and design disease gets a foot hold.

A healthy brain also requires fifteen different vitamins to function properly: B-complex, B1, B2, B6, B12, C, D, E, F, Choline, Folic Acid, Inositol, Niacin, Pantothenic Acid and Pangamic Acid = 15. Now, notice how many of the vitamins are related to or part of the B complex family, a total of eleven.

"Provided one has the correct level of vitamin, mineral and nutritional input, the body can overcome disease." –Linus Pauling, the only two time solo Nobel Prize winner.

There are foods that we eat, illicit and legal drugs that we take daily that rob the body of nutrients, refined and processed sugars rob's your body B vitamins. Sugar contains no nutrients, but it requires nutrients to metabolize sugar. Also, just as important: "Meat contains a substance that impairs brain activity and lacks a substance that the brain needs to function well." Arachidonic acid inhibits [choline] uptake, J.Neurochem 1988Apr; 50(4):1309-1318 Arachidonic acid found in meat impairs optimal functioning of the brain center for wisdom, judgment and foresight - the frontal lobe. Other milder forms of vitamin B

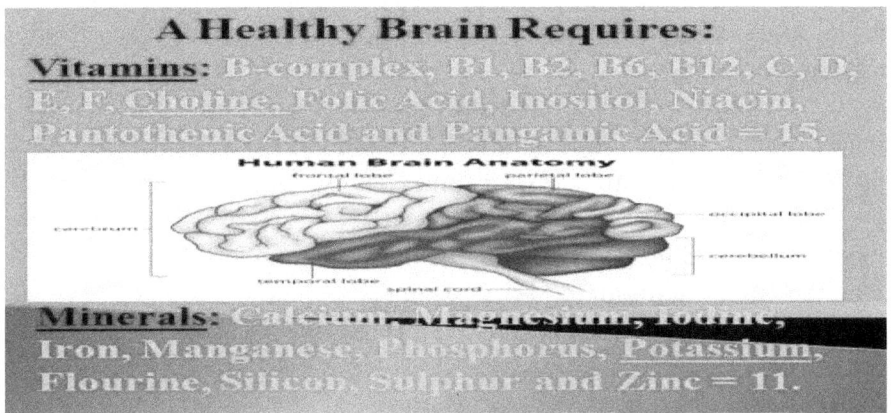

deficiencies include pernicious anemia, pellagra, beriberi, digestive disorders, poor appetite, tongue (cracks, shiny, or purple), memory loss and confusion, cardiovascular disorders, weight loss, dull and loss of hair, skin disorders, depression, fatigue, canker sores, itchy and burning eyes, and eczema (especially around genitalia area).

Many prescription drugs deplete nutrients from the body, and this is one of the reasons you need to take a nutritional supplement.

Drugs that Deplete B Vitamins

B vitamins are your best protection against elevated levels of homocysteine, an amino acid produced in the body that in excess, can increase your risk of mood disorders, poor mental performance, and Alzheimer's disease.

A wide range of drugs, from aspirin to estrogen to diuretics to stomach acid suppressors (such as Nexium and Prilosec) can interfere with the metabolism of one or more B vitamins, which can result in elevated levels of homocysteine. You who are worried about preserving your brain power, take note: medical research now clearly links poor performance on mental function tests to elevated homocysteine levels. Having too much of this amino acid floating around in your blood- stream can cost you a few IQ points! B vitamins are also critical for mood and concentration, and a severe deficiency in B vitamins (especially vitamin B12 can result in symptoms such as severe confusion and mental fog at any age. Elevated levels of homocysteine and/or low levels of B vitamins can also increase the risk of depression, stroke, Alzheimer's disease, vascular dementia, heart disease, and even certain types of cancer. If you are using a drug that depletes your body of B vitamins, you must take supplemental B vitamins daily and demand to have your homocysteine levels checked periodically by your doctor.

Pain Relievers

- Generic name: Aspirin (acetylsalicylic acid). Brand Names: Pure aspirin is sold under numerous brand names, including many private store labels. Percodan and Empirin are combination aspirin and codeine products.

Antibiotics

- Generic name: Trimethoprim: antibiotic frequently prescribed for chronic urinary tract infections. Brand Names: Bactrim, Septra

Antacid and Stomach Acid Suppressors

- Generic name: Cimetidine. Brand Names: Tagamet
- Generic name: Famotidine. Brand Names: Pepcid
- Generic name: Ranitidine. Brand Names: Zantac, Zantac 75
- Generic name: Lansoprazole. Brand Names: Prevacid
- Generic name: Nizatidine. Brand Names: Axid
- Generic name: Omeprazole. Brand Names: Prilosec

Antidiabetic Drugs

- Generic name: Metformin. Brand Names: Glucophage

Asthma Drugs
- Generic name: Beclomethasone, Brand Name: Vanceril
- Generic name: Budesonide (oral inhaler). Brand Name: Pulmacort
- Generic name: Budesonide (nasal inhaler). Brand Name: Rhinocort
- Generic name: Flunisolide (nasal inhaler). Brand Name: Nasalide
- Generic name: Flunisolide (oral inhaler). Brand Name: Aerobid
- Generic name: Fluticasone (oral inhaler). Brand Name: Flovent
- Generic name: Mometasone (nasal inhaler). Brand Name: Nasonex
- Generic name: Triamcinolone (oral inhaler). Brand Name: Azmacort
- Generic name: Theophylline. Brand Name: Aerolate

Blood Pressure-Lowering Drugs
- Generic name: Bumetanide. Brand Name: Bumex
- Generic name: Hydroclorothiazide (HCTZ), used alone or in combination with other drugs. Brand Names: Aldactazide, Capozide, Combipres, Dyazide, HydroDIURIL, Hyzaar, Lopressor-HCT, Lotensin HCT, Maxide, Microzide, Moduretic, Prinzide, Vaseretic, Zestoretic.
- Generic name: Triamterene. Brand Name: Dyrenium, or in combination with other drugs in Maxide and Dyazide.
- Generic name: Furosemide. Brand Name: Lasix
- Generic name: Hydralazine. Brand Name: Apresoline
- Generic name: Torsemide. Brand Name: Demadex

Anticonvulsant Drugs
- Generic name: Carbamazepine. Brand Name: Tegretol
- Generic name: Ethosuximide. Brand Name: Zarontin
- Generic name: Fosphenytoin. Brand Name: Cerebyx
- Generic name: Mephobarbital. Brand Name: Mebaral
- Generic name: Phenobarbital. Brand Name: Phenobarbital
- Generic name: Phenytoin. Brand Name: Dilantin
- Generic name: Primidone. Brand Name: Mysoline
- Generic name: Valproic Acid. Brand Name: Depakote, Depakene

Cholesterol-Lowering Drugs
- Generic name: Cholestyramine. Brand Name: Colestid

Estrogens
There are dozens of different brands of estrogen products, and I have only listed the major brands here. If you are taking estrogen in the form of birth control pills or hormone replacement therapy, even if you don't see your particular estrogen drug on the list, assume that it works just like any other estrogen and that you need to compensate for the loss of B vitamins by taking additional B vitamins.

- Generic name: Estrogens (with or without progesterone) as contraceptives, oral or skin patch. Brand Names: Ortho-Novum, Ortho Tri-Cyclen, Ovral, Ovcon, Demulen, Loestrin (any estrogen-containing oral contraceptive.)
- Generic name: Estrogens (with or without progesterone) for hormone replacement therapy for menopause or hysterectomy; oral, skin patch, or cream. Brand Names: Premarin, Prempro, Activela, Combinpatch, Estrotest, any hormone replacement product containing estrogen.

Estrogen Substitutes for Osteoporosis
- Generic name: Raloxifene. Brand Name: Evista

Anti-Parkinson's Drugs
- Generic name: Carbidopa and levodopa. Brand Name: Sinemet
 Nonsteroidal Antiinflammatory Drugs (NSAIDS)
- Generic name: Celecoxib. Brand Name: Celebrex
- Generic name: Ibuprofen. Brand Name: Advil, Bayer Select, Motrin, Midol, etc.
- Generic name: Indomethacin. Brand Name: Indocin
- Generic name: Naproxen. Brand Name: Naprosyn, Aleve, etc.

Corticosteroids
Anti-inflammatory Drugs Used to treat asthma, arthritis, allergy, and pain.
- Generic name: Methyl Prednisolone. Brand Name: Medrol
- Generic name: Prednisone. Brand Name: Deltasone, Orasone

- -drperlmutter.com/learn/resources/drugs-that-deplete-b-vitamins

With the processed, manufactured, and refined foods in the stores today, which I have adopted the term "man intervention foods." Along with manufactured foods high in processed and refined sugars, combined with prescription medications, we wonder why poor mental health is on the rise worldwide. The prescription drug that you are taking for one condition is causing other problems, but you already know that. The problem is that you do not have the knowledge of Naturopathy or trust the natural healing process.

Synthetic Vitamins

To add insult to injury or as my dad would say, pouring salt in to a wound; more than 95% of vitamins sold today are synthetic. They are manufactured with chemicals in a lab. You may even be taking one your doctor recommended. Unless your doctor is also a natural practitioner there is a big chance they are synthetic. Vitamins like Centrum, One a Day, etc… just about all vitamins sold in a grocery store; including your local GNC and Nature Made. An example of synthetic vitamins is a form of vitamin B12 called Cyanocobalamin. The true natural form of B12 is called Methylcobalamin. Cyanocobalamin, the synthetic form of vitamin B12 is approximately 100 times cheaper than Methylcobalamin, the all natural B12. Not only are they cheaper but they have a far longer shelf life. The following short list of companies are owned by the pharmaceutical companies: Nature Made is owned by Thai Otsuka Pharmaceutical Co, Ltd., Centrum is owned by Pfizer, One A Day is owned by Bayer, etc... Unfortunately, the majority of these supplements are not doing for your body what you believed or hoped and in fact, can result in toxic accumulation, while having a devastating effect on your health. **Synthetic calcium has** been proven to increase your risk of heart attack and stroke by as much as 30%. What about all the food that we eat that is being fortified with B vitamins, iron and calcium? All of those foods need to be able to sit on the shelves for a very long period of time. Who are you feeding them to; your children and they all have synthetic vitamins in them. There is truly a difference between all natural and synthetic. The synthetic version is really creating a toxic overload on your system, and if they are creating a toxic overload on your system; Just Think of what they are doing to your Children. Educate yourself about vitamins then find very good all-natural vitamins.

Nutriments & Micro-Nutrients

Vitamins, minerals, antioxidants, phytonutrients and trace elements are necessary to prevent any disorder and disease, resulting from any nutrient deficiency. Vitamins control the body's appropriation of minerals, and in the absence of minerals they have no function to perform. Lacking vitamins, the system can make some use of minerals, but lacking minerals, vitamins are useless.

Vitamins that focus on mood and cognition:

- B vitamins: anti stress and energy
- B1 Thiamin: helps to prevent memory loss
- B3 Niacin
- helps you relax, help you get to sleep more rapidly, can reduce anxiety and depression
- B6 regulate mood and helps to prevent mental fatigue
- B9 Foliate and Folic acid: improves cognition and memory function
- B12: helps in the metabolism of energy and helps maintain the central nervous system
- D3: the sunshine vitamin, it improves memory
    - Low levels associated with depression, dementia, cognitive decline and Alzheimer's

- Iron: is for concentration, attention, focus, beneficial effect on mood
- Magnesium is the calming and relaxing micronutrient, it helps with concentration and focus, better sleep, helps you relax and get into a better mood, it reduces cravings, reduces anxiety and helps you cope with stress, which makes it good for ADHD and hyperactivity
- Zinc: is the male mineral but woman need it to, the highest amount is in the brain. Its helps with the body and brain's ability to handle stress
    - Low levels are linked to depression
- Vitamin E protects against neuronal degeneration and slow rate of cognitive decline.

God's plan is to educate v. man's plan which is to medicate. Let's utilize the Eight Doctors and food supplementation first.

- Calcium is another micronutrient that plays a role in reducing stress, relaxation and has a calming effect,
- Vitamin C protects the brain from free radicals
- Potassium supports memory function and stress reduction
- Many mental health disorders such as depression, anxiety, bi-polar, *Schizophreni,* ADHD, Autisum, OCD, are all associated with nutrient deficiencies

Let's look at nutrition before we medicate. Obviously, if someone is the threat or danger to himself or others then we must help that individual medically.

Drs. Water, Oxygen and Sleep are all nutrients that are good for the brain.

- Our nervous system is the primary communication system in our body.
- It is a network of neurons of approximately 100 billion that connect organs to the brain.
- Neurotransmitters are the chemicals in the brain that regulate mood and emotions.
- Serotonin and Norepinephine are two neurotransmitters that are involved with depression, mood and other psychiatric disorders.

Brain Chemicals that Regulate Mood

- Serotonin is the feel good neurotransmitter (N.T.) it requires L-Tryptophan
    - Dopamine is the reward and pleasure center – L-Tyrosine
    - Norepinephrine for energy, alert, concentration and focus - L-Tyrosine
    - Glutamate supports excitatory, learning and memory

- Acetylcholine helps to induce Rapid Eye Movement (REM) sleep
- GABA reduces inhibition and regulates anxiety

It is a fact the recent research suggests that over 90% of your body's serotonin is produced in the gut (intestinal flora). This is one more reason why the digestive system is so important to human health. Although serotonin is well known as a brain neurotransmitter, <u>it is estimated that 90 percent of the body's serotonin is made in the digestive tract</u>. New research at Caltech, published in the April 9 issue of the journal *Cell*, <u>shows that certain bacteria in the gut are important for the production of peripheral serotonin</u>.
http://www.caltech.edu/news/microbes-help-produce-serotonin-gut-46495

SSRI's and SNRI's

SSRI's or <u>selective serotonin reuptake inhibitors</u> and SNRIs, <u>serotonin and Norepinephrine reuptake inhibitors</u> do not actually increase the amount of serotonin molecules in the brain. SSRI's are thought to block the re-absorption (reuptake) of serotonin by certain nerve cells in the brain. This theoretically leaves more serotonin available in the brain. However if you have low serotonin to begin with these medications either will not work well, or work for a while then "poop out". The claims of Big Pharma that the <u>SSRI drugs</u> increase serotonin levels in the brain is really only a clever partial truth (a plausible "white lie"). In actuality, SSRI drugs only temporarily and momentarily increase the levels of serotonin in the gap between serotonin nerves (called the "synapse") while – long term – they actually decrease and wasting the stored-up serotonin in the pre-synaptic nerves. The serotonin is actually depleted by the SSRIs well-advertised and, at the same time, poorly explained function: the inhibiting (= disabling) of the reuptake pump's physiologically normal recycling of the neurotransmitter back into the pre-synaptic nerve, which allows repeated reuse of the same serotonin molecules for future nerve impulse transmission. Thus, the unadvertised result of repeated inhibition of the reuptake mechanism is the long-term depletion (and destruction by synaptic enzyme systems) of serotonin directly because of the drug's major mechanism of action. This depletion of stored-up serotonin helps to explain the phenomenon of "Prozac Poop-Out" which commonly results in the need to increase the dosage of an SSRI to obtain the same artificially stimulating effect or to avoid the common withdrawal symptoms that happen when the drug is stopped abruptly, the dose decreased or the synapse function altered and/or damaged. Patients on any number of prescription or illicit brain-altering drugs commonly develop withdrawal symptoms by just staying on the (increasingly ineffective) initial dose (a "poop-out" phenomenon also known as "tolerance"). Tolerance happens with the regular use of dependency-inducing drugs such as dopamine -norepinephrine reuptake inhibitor psychostimulants such as cocaine, the amphetamines (including Adderall), methamphetamine, Ecstasy, Effexor, Wellbutrin and the cocaine-like drug Ritalin) or the GABA agonists such as the tranquilizers/anti-anxiety drugs/hypnotics/sleeping pills such as Valium, Xanax, Klonopin, Restoril, Ambien, Lunesta, etc. This depletion of stored-up serotonin helps to explain the phenomenon of "Prozac Poop-Out" which commonly results in the need to increase the dosage of an SSRI to obtain the same artificially stimulating effect or to avoid the common withdrawal symptoms that happen when the drug is stopped abruptly, the dose decreased or the synapse function altered and/or damaged.

  Patients on any number of prescription or illicit brain-altering drugs commonly develop withdrawal symptoms by just staying on the (increasingly ineffective) initial dose (a "poop-out" phenomenon also known as "tolerance"). Tolerance happens with the regular use of dependency-inducing drugs such as dopamine/norepinephrine reuptake inhibitor psychostimulants such as cocaine, the amphetamines (including Adderall), methamphetamine, Ecstasy, Effexor, Wellbutrin and the cocaine-like drug Ritalin) or the GABA agonists such as the tranquilizers/anti-anxiety drugs/hypnotics/sleeping pills such as Valium, Xanax, Klonopin, Restoril, Ambien, Lunesta, etc.

  "Prescription drugs are emergency medicine for immediate life threatening events, long term use contributes to the health problem. The Physiological System adapts to each medication and shortly thereafter the tranquilizers act upon the system as stimulants, and the anti-depressants like depressants after prolonged use." Elden M. Chalmers Ph.D. Healing the Broken Brain, p. 55, 56.

"Prolonged use of prescription drugs tends to make a condition worse." Dr. Dean Black, Health Care at the Crossroads, p. 29. So it is the best interest of the patient to stabilize themselves and have their medical doctor or psychiatrist work with a Naturopathic doctor, not just a nutritionist or dietitian. For true healing to take place, "the patient must enlist the powers of appropriate thinking to bring about true healing." Elden M. Chalmers Ph.D. Healing the Broken Brain, p. 55, 56.

Natural Serotonin Supplements

Natural serotonin supplements are likely to be the most effective means to raise serotonin levels in the brain while being safe and without the side effects of anti depression medications. 5-HTP, or 5-hydroxy tryptophan, is a safe dietary supplement that introduces higher levels of tryptophan into the blood stream, which then enters the central nervous system and facilitate the needed synthesis of serotonin. But the important issue of this book (especially for people who want to take control of their own emotional and mental health issues) is that synthetic brain-altering drugs, which are all lethal at a certain dose (as opposed to the benign and healthy neurotransmitter precursors), never, never cure mental ill health. At best, they only mask symptoms that are often misinterpreted as representing "mental illnesses". Indeed, neurological dysfunction caused by psychotropic drugs is almost universal. These unintended adverse effects commonly cause symptoms that mimic mental illnesses. (See the extensive lists of adverse neurotoxic and psychotoxic "adverse" effects of any prescription psych drug in the dispensing pharmacy's product insert or in the PDR [Physician's Desk Reference] to confirm this reality for yourself). Amino acid therapy for a variety of emotional issues has been proven to be an important adjunct in the cure of uncounted numbers of patients fortunate enough to know about brain nutrient therapy before getting on drugs.

Again, it is important to reiterate that serotonin can only be increased in the brain (or body, since 90% of the serotonin in the body is in the intestinal system – accounting for the many gastro-intestinal "side effects" caused by the SSRI drugs) by eating the proper food or supplementing the diet with the amino acid supplements L-Tryptophan and/or 5-HTP, along with various co-factors that facilitate the metabolic process in the serotonin brain cell's manufacturing process. Adequate amounts of these co-factors are best obtained by taking therapeutic doses of magnesium, zinc, folic acid, vitamins C and B6. Unfortunately, of the amino acids in the protein foods we humans commonly consume, tryptophan is the scarcest one of them all. The proteins that contain the most tryptophan include white meat, dairy protein, beans, egg whites, pumpkin seeds, sunflower seeds, peanuts, lentils and bananas. The amounts of tryptophan in those foods still contain only a fraction of what are found in the dietary supplements L-Tryptophan and 5-HTP. As an example, it would take 100 grams of pumpkin seeds to yield the brain serotonin that could be derived from one 500 mg capsule of tryptophan or one 50 mg capsule of 5-HTP. It needs to be noted that this basic brain science report about holistic mental health is for informational purposes only and is not meant to be a prescription for any given person, especially for people who are already taking psychotropic drugs.

It needs to be noted that this basic brain science report about holistic mental health is for informational purposes only and is not meant to be a prescription for any given person, especially for people who are already taking psychotropic drugs. For patients who want further information concerning dosages of the mentioned supplements, they should consult a nutritionally-oriented Naturopathic doctor, and/or health practitioner, or books such as Depression-Free for Life (Cousens), Prescription for Nutritional Healing (Balch), 5-HTP: Nature's Serotonin Solution or Mind Boosters (both by Sahelian), Heal With Amino Acids (Sahley and Birkner), The Mood Cure (Ross), among others. For advice on information about the toxicity of, and the problems concerning withdrawal from, psychotropic drugs, it is advised that people read books such as Prozac Backlash and The Antidepressant Solution (both by Glenmullen), Your Drug May Be Your Problem, Medication Madness and Toxic Psychiatry (all by Breggin), Madness in America: Bad Science, Bad Medicine and the Maltreatment of the Mentally Ill (Whitaker).

"As it turns out, there are alternative medical treatments for depression. Foremost among these is L-Tryptophan, a critical amino acid the body cannot manufacture for itself. Both L-Tryptophan and Prozac work with serotonin, a chemical that has to do with how we feel." "Elevated levels of serotonin in the body often result in the relief of depression, as well as substantial reduction in pain sensitivity, anxiety and stress. Prozac, as well as other new anti-depressant drugs such as Paxil and Zoloft, attempt to enhance levels of serotonin by working on whatever amounts of it already exist in the body (these drugs are known as selective serotonin reuptake inhibitors). None of these drugs, however, produce serotonin. In contrast, ingested L-Tryptophan acts to produce serotonin, even in individuals who generate little serotonin of their own. The most effective way to elevate levels of serotonin would be to use a serotonin producer rather than a serotonin enhancer." Dean Wolfe Manders, Ph.D. "Thus it is clear that L-Tryptophan and Prozac are in competition with each other. Prozac is a drug that fools the body and L-Tryptophan is an amino acid that creates more serotonin. Prozac, and similar drugs, have been shown to have deadly side-effects. But I won't get into that."

Another cold hard reality is pharmaceutical drugs especially when consumed to manage chronic disease and symptoms cause severe side effects that also damage, harm and kill. The most prescribed drugs of all are painkillers that typically are highly addictive. Big Pharma with the help of their global army of doctors have purposely and calculatingly turned a large percentage of us especially in the United States into hardcore drug addicts, both physically and [psychologically] addicted to artificial synthetic substances that are detrimental to our health and well-being. More than three quarters of US citizens over 50 are currently taking prescribed medication. One in four women in their 40's and 50's is taking [antidepressants]. Though the US contains just 5% of the world population, it consumes over half of all prescribed medication and a phenomenal 80% of the world's supply of painkillers. Those who admit to taking prescription drugs on average take four different prescription drugs daily. Taking massive amounts of prescription drugs has caused an epidemic that's part of a sinister plan to squeeze yet more profit out of a system designed to keep humans chronically unhealthy.

The Food and Drug Administration (FDA)

To better understand why pharmaceuticals like Prozac are pushed upon the public and natural treatments are ruthlessly suppressed, you have to understand the role and who funds the FDA.

"There has been many cancer cures, and all have been ruthlessly and systematically suppressed with a Gestapo-like thoroughness by the cancer establishment…" Robert C. Atkins, M.D.

One has to wonder, if they would suppress natural cancer cures, they would surely do it with other natural treatments for disease. The Food and Drug Administration is a federal agency of the United States Department of Health and Human Services, one of the United States federal executive departments. Wikipedia.

"The FDA is largely controlled by the orthodox medical profession… and the industries which the FDA was set up to regulate." –Miles Robinson, M.D., Head of a Congressional Committee investigating allegations of a conspiracy to suppress alternative therapies.

"The FDA is serving industry rather than the public." Dr. David Graham, Senior drug safety researcher at the FDA who blew the whistle on Vioxx.

"The thing that bugs me the most is that people think the FDA is protecting them. It isn't. What the FDA is doing and what the public thinks its doing are as different as night and day." Herbert Lay, former Commissioner of the FDA.

The BMJ was formally the British Medical Journal covered the FDA on Nov. 19, 2003 - The cover photo of the September 14 BMJ, in which this article first appeared, showed the FDA building in Rockville, Maryland, above the provocative caption, "Who owns the FDA?" A news report in that issue quoted a former FDA consultant: "[*the agency has become] a servant of the industry, where dissenting voices are intimidated and ostracized*" (*BMJ* 2002;325:561). www.bmj.com/content/327/7418/E160

Big Pharma's top eleven corporations generated net profits in just one decade from 2003 to 2012 of nearly three quarters of a trillion dollars – that's just net profit alone. The net profit for 2012 amongst those top eleven amounted to $85 billion in just that one year. The majority of these largest pharmaceuticals are headquartered in the US – including the top four, Johnson & Johnson (#39 on Fortune 500 list), Pfizer (#51), Merck (#65) and Eli Lilly (#129) along with Abbott (#152) and Bristol Myer Squibb (#176). 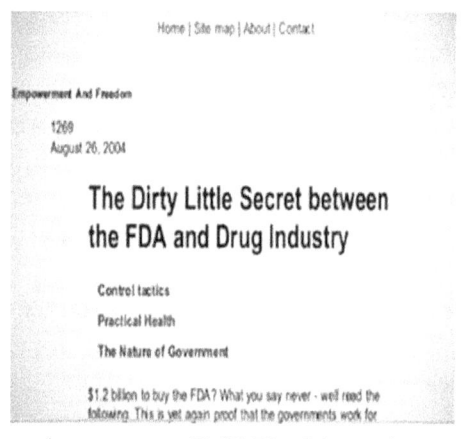 The healthcare research company IMS Health projects worldwide sales of Pharma drugs to exceed one trillion dollars by 2014. With that kind of obscenely powerful money to throw around, what Big Pharma wants, Big Pharma nearly always gets. Just as the oligarchs buy, own and control national governments to do their sleazy bidding, Big Pharma as an extension of those same oligarchs does too. Perhaps what makes Big Pharma unique in the US is that the industry outspends all others in laying down cold hard cash into its lobbying efforts – another word for bribing governments that includes not only US Congress (and parliaments) but its US federal regulator, the bought and sold Food and Drug Administration (FDA). It poured $2.7 billion into its lobbying interests from 1998 to 2013, 42% more than the second most "Gov. Corp." bribe which happens to be its sister industry insurance. And it's this unholy trinity of the medical establishment (personified by the American Medical Association), embedded insurance industry that wrote Obamacare into law and Big Pharma that makes the United States the most costly, broken, corrupt, destructive healthcare system in the entire world. The structured system is designed and layered with built in incentives at every tier to make and keep people sick, chronically dependent on their drugs for survival that merely mask and smother symptoms rather than cure or eradicate the root cause of disease.

The FDA and L-Tryptophan

Now that you understand that the FDA is protecting the Pharmeuctical Industries interest and not the public's, let see how they have limited the availability of L-Tryptophan to the health consumer.

"So what is the FDA going to do? It is deadly Prozac versus harmless and far more effective L-Tryptophan. This is what they did: In the fall of 1989, the FDA recalled L-Tryptophan, an amino acid nutritional supplement, stating that it caused a rare and deadly flu-like condition (Eosinophilia-Myalgia Syndrome — EMS). On March 22, 1990, the FDA banned the public sale of dietary L-Tryptophan completely. This ban continues today." (Ed. Note: The ban was eventually lifted about a decade later.) On March 26, 1990, Newsweek featured a lead article praising the virtues of the anti-depressant drug Prozac. Its multi-color cover displayed a floating, gigantic green and white capsule of Prozac with the caption: "Prozac: A Breakthrough Drug for Depression."

"The fact that the FDA ban of L-Tryptophan and the Newsweek magazine Prozac cover story occurred within four days of each other went unnoticed by both the media and the public. Yet, to those who understand the effective properties of L-Tryptophan and Prozac, the concurrence seems unbelievably coincidental. The link here is the brain neurotransmitter serotonin — a biochemical nerve signal conductor. The action of Prozac and L-Tryptophan are both involved with serotonin, but in totally different ways." "You need to understand that it takes far more than 4 days to get an issue of Newsweek magazine out the door. Thus, the magazine was working on the Prozac article weeks before the FDA issued their order. You should also understand that the FDA did not prove that L-Tryptophan was dangerous. They banned it because a drug company issued a contaminated batch of L-Tryptophan." "Normally, when a drug company issues a bad batch of a product, which is quite common, the FDA fines the company and may have some other punishment for the company. But the FDA does not ban the product! But in this case the FDA banned the harmless and useful product. It's a real crime competing with Big Pharma. This "double standard" is standard operating procedure for the totally corrupt FDA. Thus we have a situation where Congress has allowed for several decades for tobacco products to be manufactured and sold, which are known to kill hundreds of thousands of Americans every year, but at the same time Congress has allowed the FDA to ban L-Tryptophan."

"The public availability of L-Tryptophan is too important an issue only to be argued and shrouded within a scientific debate that remains,

ultimately, mystifying to the vast majority of Americans. There are many obvious facts worthy of public attention, and public concern. For example, consider the following: On February 9, 1993, a United States government patent (#5185157) was issued to use L-Tryptophan to treat, and cure EMS, the very same deadly flu-like condition which prompted the FDA to take L-Tryptophan off the market in 1989. Notwithstanding its public ban and import alert on
L-Tryptophan, the FDA today allows Ajinomoto U.S.A. the right to
Import from Japan human-use L-Tryptophan. Distributed from the Ajinomoto plant in Raleigh, North Carolina, the L-Tryptophan is then sold to, and through, a network of compounding pharmacies across the United States. Purchased by individuals only under a physician's order, L-Tryptophan emerges as a new prescription drug in the serotonin marketplace in one hundred, 500 mg capsules costing about $75 — approximately five times more than if they were sold as a dietary supplement.

    Since the FDA holds the political mandate and power of a public regulatory agency established, ostensibly, to protect people from raw corporate interests in drug production and distribution, the actions of the FDA in concert with Ajinomoto U.S.A. are illuminating. By publicly banning L-Tryptophan from its dietary supplement status and price, while allowing L-Tryptophan to be sold as a high-priced prescription drug, the naked duplicity of FDA L-Tryptophan policy is revealed. During and after the 1989 EMS outbreak, the FDA did not totally ban the use of L-Tryptophan in humans — then, as today, the FDA has granted the pharmaceutical industry the protected right to use L-Tryptophan in hospital settings. Manufactured by Abbott Laboratories, the amino acid injectable solutions Aminosyn and Aminosyn II contain as much as 200 mg of L-Tryptophan. (Moreover, L-Tryptophan has never been removed from baby food produced and sold within the United States.)

    "While the FDA has banned the public sale and use of the safe,
non-contaminated, dietary supplement L-Tryptophan for people, the United States Department of Agriculture still sanctions the legal sale and use of non-contaminated L-Tryptophan for animals. Today, as in the past, feed grade L-Tryptophan continues to be used as a nutritional and bulk feed additive by the commercial hog and chicken farming industry. Additionally, L-Tryptophan is now available for use by veterinarians in caring for horses and pets. Outside of the United States, in countries such as Canada, the Netherlands, Germany, England, and others, L-Tryptophan is widely used. Nowhere, have any serious or widespread health problems

occurred." ihealthtube.com/content/only-two-ways-raise-brain-serotonin-levels.

The below article From the FDA.gov website sheds more light on precautions the public can take since the FDA lifted the ban on L-Tryptophan in 2005.

Post-epidemic eosinophilia myalgia syndrome associated with L-Tryptophan

Jeffrey A Allen,[1] Alicia Peterson,[2] Robert Sufit,[1] Monique E Hinchcliff,[2] J. Matthew Mahoney,[4] Tammara A Wood,[4] Frederick W Miller,[3] Michael L Whitfield,[4] and John Varga*[2]

Introduction

Eosinophilia–myalgia syndrome (EMS), a chronic multisystem disorder first recognized in 1989, is characterized by sub acute onset of myalgias and peripheral eosinophilia associated with chronic muscle, nerve, fascia, and skin involvement.[1,2] This apparently new disease occurred in an epidemic outbreak that over a 6-month period affected 1,500 individuals and was associated with over 30 deaths.[3] The Centers for Disease Control (CDC) proposed a surveillance case definition of EMS that included peripheral blood eosinophilia and severe generalized myalgias.[4] Toxico-epidemiologic studies linked EMS to L-tryptophan (L-TRP) containing dietary supplements manufactured using genetically-engineered bacteria.[5] Initial analysis of implicated L-TRP revealed an impurity that was identified as 1'1'-ethylidenebis [tryptophan] (EBT).[6] Removal of L-TRP from the market was followed by swift resolution of the EMS epidemic.

The pathobiological basis of EMS remains unknown. Epidemiologic studies tracing implicated L-TRP to a single manufacturer and quantitative analyses of EBT suffered from methodological limitations. EBT was just one of more than 60 minor impurities detected in implicated L-TRP, six of which were associated with EMS.[7] One of these, 3-(phenylamino)alanine (PAA), shares chemical properties with 3-(N-phenylamino)-1,2-propanediol (PAP) that was implicated in the 1981 Spanish toxic oil syndrome (TOS) epidemic linked to consumption of aniline-denatured rapeseed oil.[8]

The FDA lifted the ban on L-TRP in 2005, allowing L-TRP-containing products to again be available as dietary supplements. Since that time it has been recognized that some individuals possess putative immunogenetic risk and protective factors for EMS.[12] We report the first new case, to our knowledge, of L-TRP-associated EMS occurring since the reintroduction of L-TRP… Immunostaining with antibodies to the eosinophil degranulation products major basic protein (MBP) and eosinophil-derived neurotoxin (EDN) were strongly positive (Figs. 2 H,I). HLA-DR typing revealed that the patient had the HLA-DRB1*04 allele, <u>a risk factor among L-TRP users for the development of EMS</u> (OR 3.9, 95% CI 1.1–16.4), and the <u>absence of any of the reported protective HLA alleles</u>.[12]

Instead of banning pure uncontaminated L-tryptophan from the public market place, since the product that caused the EMS outbreak was contaminated, allow individuals that have concerns to be tested to see if they have the <u>HLA-DRB1*04 allele</u> and/or <u>protective HLA alleles</u>.

References

1. Hertzman PA, Blevins WL, Mayer J, Greenfield B, Ting M, Gleich GJ. Association of the eosinophilia-myalgia syndrome with the ingestion of tryptophan. N Engl J Med. 1990;322:869–73. [PubMed]
2. Silver RM, Heyes MP, Maize JC, Quearry B, Vionnet-Fuasset M, Sternberg EM. Scleroderma, fasciitis, and eosinophilia associated with the ingestion of tryptophan. N Engl J Med. 1990;322:874–81. [PubMed]
3. Swygert LA, Back EE, Auerbach SB, Sewell LE, Falk H. Eosinophilia-myalgia syndrome: mortality data from the US national surveillance system. J Rheumatol. 1993;20:1711–17. [PubMed]
4. Eosinophilia-myalgia syndrome and L-tryptophan-containing products--New Mexico, Minnesota, Oregon, and New York, 1989. Centers for Disease Control (CDC) MMWR Morb Mortal Wkly Rep. 1989;38:785–8. [PubMed]
5. Belongia EA, Hedberg CW, Gleich GJ, et al. An investigation of the cause of the eosinophilia-myalgia syndrome associated with tryptophan use. N Engl J Med. 1990;323:357–65. [PubMed]
6. Mayeno AN, Lin F, Foote CS, et al. Characterization of "peak E," a novel amino acid associated with eosinophilia-myalgia syndrome. Science. 1990;250:1707– [PubMed].
7. Hill RH, Jr, Caudill SP, Philen RM, et al. Contaminants in L-tryptophan associated with eosinophilia myalgia syndrome. Arch Environ Contam Toxicol. 1993;25:134–42. [PubMed]
8. Mayeno AN, Belongia EA, Lin F, Lundy SK, Gleich GJ. 3-(Phenylamino)alanine, a novel aniline-derived amino acid associated with the eosinophilia-myalgia syndrome: a link to the toxic oil syndrome? Mayo Clin Proc. 1992;67:1134–
12. Okada S, Kamb ML, Pandey JP, Philen RM, Love LA, Miller FW. Immunogenetic risk and protective factors for the development of L-tryptophan-associated eosinophilia-myalgia syndrome and associated symptoms. Arthritis Rheum. 2009;61:1305–11. [PMC free article] [PubMed].

Griffonia Simplicifolia (5-HTP)

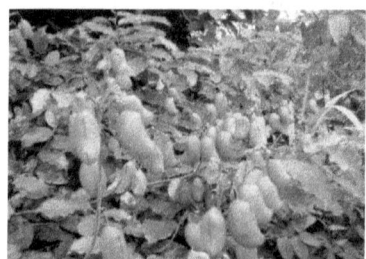

Compounds:
Griffonia contains several indole derivatives including 5-Hydroxy-L-tryptophan, indole-acetylaspartic acid and 5hydroxy indole-3-acetic acid (5-HIAA).

Effects:
5-Hydroxtryptophan (5-HTP) is the intermediate metabolite of the amino acid L-tryptophan (LT) in the serotonin pathway. Therapeutic use of 5-HTP bypasses the conversion of LT into 5-HTP by the enzyme tryptophan hydrolase, which is the rate limiting step in the synthesis of serotonin. Tryptophan hydrolase can be inhibited by numerous factors, including stress, insulin resistance, vitamin B6 deficiency, and insufficient magnesium. In addition, these same factors can increase the conversion of LT to kynurenine via tryptophan oxygenase, making LT unavailable for serotonin production. Tryptophan hydrolase and kynurenine levels are factors to have evaluated before Taking antipsychotic drugs. 5-HTP functions as an antioxidant; whereas LT can actually promote oxidative damage. 5-HTP is well absorbed from an oral dose, with about 70% ending up in the bloodstream. Absorption of 5-HTP is not affected by the presence of other amino acids; therefore it may be taken with meals without reducing its effectiveness. Unlike LT, 5-HTP cannot be shunted into niacin or protein production. Serotonin levels in the brain are highly dependent on levels of 5-HTP and LT in the central nervous system (CNS). 5-HTP easily crosses the blood-brain barrier, not requiring the presence of a transport molecule with several other amino acids, the presence of these competing amino acids can inhibit LT transport into the brain. 5-HTP acts primarily by increasing levels of serotonin within the CNS. The other neurotransmitters and CNS chemicals, such as melatonin, dopamine, norepinephrine, and beta-endorphin, have also been shown to increase following oral administration of 5-HTP.

Clinical trials: Depression

To date, some 40 studies have evaluated the clinical effects of 5-HTP on depression. In an open trial design, a total of 107 patients with endogenous unipolar or bipolar were given daily oral dosages of 5-HTP from 50 to 300 mg. Significant improvement was observed in 74% of the patients (69%), and no significant side effects were reported. The response rate in most of these patients was quite rapid (less than two weeks). Speed of response was subsequently addressed in a study of 59 patients with eight different types of depression. 5- HTP was administered orally in dosages from 150 to 300 mg daily for a period of three weeks. Thirteen patients (22%) were markedly improved, and another 27 patients (45.8%) showed moderate improvement. Of these 40 patients who improved, 20 (50%) begun to show improvement within three days, and 32 patients (80%) improved within two weeks of beginning treatment with 5-HTP (Sano, 1972).

The effectiveness of 5-hydroxy-L-trytophan as an antidepressant drug was studied in 59 patients with depressive symptoms in a double blind clinical study using a Rating Scale for Depression (Nakajima, 1978). A daily dose of 150-300 mg of 5-hydroxyl-L-tryptophan was administered for three weeks. Favorable response was observed in 40 patients (67.8%), of whom 13 patients were markedly improved. These effects were observed in 32 patients (80% of the improved patients) within a week of the treatment. Analysis indicated that endogenous depression and involutional or senile depression were the preferable indications of 5-hydroxy-L-tryptophan loading. The main side effects of 5-hydroxy-L-tryptophan were gastrointestinal disturbances which were minimized by the simultaneous administration of metoclopromide or trihexphenidyl.

Employing positron-emission tomography, 8 healthy volunteers and 6 people diagnosed with major depression received infusions of radio labeled 5-HTP. Significantly less 5-HTP crossed the blood-brain barrier into the brains of the depressed subjects than into the brains of the normal controls. A significant reduction in anxiety was observed on three different scales designed to measure anxiety (Agren, 1991).

A double-blind clinical trial was carried out involving 26 hospitals, depressed patients who were randomized into two groups and received chlorimipramine (50 mg/day), combined with L-5-HTP (300 mg/day) in Group A, and with placebo in Group B. For 28 days, patients were evaluated by Hamilton rating Scale for Depression (HRSD) each week; and by ZDIS and CGI at the beginning and end of treatment. The results for both types of pathology were quantitatively and qualitatively more positive for Group A than for Group B (Nardini, 1983).

5-HTP was administered to 24 patients hospitalized for depression. After two weeks of treatment, amelioration of depressive systems was observed in seven patients diagnosed with unipolar depression. A 30% increase in the levels of 5-hydroxyindolacetic acid, the primary metabolite of serotonin, was also noted in the patients' cerebrospinal fluid. This suggests that the exogenous 5-HTP was converted to serotonin within the central nervous system (takahashi, 1975).

5-HTP was evaluated in comparison to a Selective Serotonin Reuptake Inhibitor (SSRI) drug in a double-blind, multicenter study design (Poldinger, 1991). A total of 36 subjects, all of whom were diagnosed with some form of depression, received either 100 mg of 5-HTP three times per day, or 150 mg of fluvoxamine (an SSRI) three times daily. The subjects were evaluated at 0, 2, 4, and 6 weeks, using four evaluation tools: the Hamilton Rating Scale for Depression (HRSD), a standard depression rating scale; a patient-performed self-assessment; the investigator's assessment of severity; and a global clinical impression. Both treatment groups showed significant and nearly equal reduction in depression beginning in week two and continuing through week six. After four weeks, 15 of the 36 patients treated with 5-HTP, and 18 of the 33 patients treated with fluvoxamine had improved by at least 50 percent, according to the HRSD scores. By week six, the two groups had about equal numbers showing 50 percent improvement. When the numbers were totaled at the end of the study, researchers found the mean percentage improvement from baseline to the final assessment was slightly greater for patients treated 5-HTP. The number of treatment failures was higher in the fluvoxamine group (5/29, 17%) than in the 5-HTP group (2/34. 6%), although neither of these differences were statistically significant. All four evaluation tools yielded similar results. The study also looked at the incidence of adverse effects from both treatments, which were found to be rare and generally mild, usually occurring during the first few days of treatment and then disappearing. Overall, 5-HTP appeared to be slightly better tolerated than fluvoxamine, although the results did not reach the level of statistical significant. Tolerance was assessed as being "good to very good" in 34/36 patients receiving 5-HTP (94.5%), compared to 28/33 in the fluvoxamine group (84.8%). 5-HTP has also been compared in a few studies with conventional tricyclic antidepressants (chloripramine and imipramine)-the most effective drugs for treating depression until the development of the SSRIs.

–Physician Desk Reference for Herbal Medicines, Fourth Edition, section Herbal Monographs, p. 3, 4.

When I go to the Webmed website, the list of possible side effects is more telling than the results mentioned above.

Side Effects: Nausea, vomiting, drowsiness, dizziness, loss of appetite, **depressed mood**, trouble sleeping, weakness, and sweating may occur. <u>If any of these effects persist or worsen</u>, tell your doctor or pharmacist promptly.

Tell your doctor right away if you have any serious side effects, including: easy bruising/bleeding, shaking (tremor), and decrease in sexual interest/ability.

Get medical help right away if you have any very serious side effects, including: fainting, black stools, vomit that looks like coffee grounds, seizures, eye pain/swelling/redness, widened pupils, vision changes (such as seeing rainbows around lights at night, blurred vision).

This medication may increase serotonin and rarely cause a very serious condition called serotonin syndrome/toxicity. The risk increases if you are also taking other drugs that increase serotonin, so tell your doctor or pharmacist of all the drugs you take (see Drug Interactions section). Get medical help right away if you develop some of the following symptoms: fast heartbeat, hallucinations, loss of coordination, severe dizziness, severe nausea/vomiting/diarrhea, twitching muscles, unexplained fever, and unusual restlessness.

Rarely, males may have a painful or prolonged erection lasting 4 or more hours. If this occurs, stop using this drug and get medical help right away, or permanent problems could occur.

A very serious allergic reaction to this drug is rare. However, get medical help right away if you notice any symptoms of a serious allergic reaction, including: rash, itching/swelling (especially of the face/tongue/throat), severe dizziness, trouble breathing.

This is not a complete list of possible side effects. If you notice other effects not listed above, contact your doctor or pharmacist.

In the US -

Call your doctor for medical advice about side effects. You may report side effects to FDA at 1-800-FDA-1088 or at www.fda.gov/medwatch.

In Canada - Call your doctor for medical advice about side effects. You may report side effects to Health Canada at 1-866-234-2345.

https://www.webmd.com/drugs/2/drug-1049-7095/fluvoxamine-oral/fluvoxamine-oral/details

The disclaimer below is very telling as medical doctors, psychiatrist, pediatricians, etc… are willing to subject their patients to side effects and some life threatening, instead of trying a natural approach first.

Remember that your doctor has prescribed this medication because he or she has judged that the benefit to you is greater than the risk of side effects. Many people using this medication do not have serious side effects.

    The second thing that jumps out at me is that the above clinical trials proved that 5-HTP slightly outperformed the SSRIs, with no statistical difference in adverse reactions then why not give their patients the option of trying natural protocols first?

    Finally, the clinical trials, double blind studies I referenced to above were all conducted before or at the beginning of the FDA band on all sales of 5-HTP on March 22, 1990; and was not reinstated until 2005. How many clinical trials do you think took place while the FDA's ban was in place? During this fifteen year period, how many psychiatrist, medical doctors, psychologist, pediatricians, etc… were taught the benefits of 5-HTP? When you combine the above information with the startling fact that a term "chemical imbalance" is a made up phrase that cannot be measured by a blood test, PET or CAT, urine test or any other standardized medical test then you have to start thinking outside the box and search for a psychologist or psychiatrist like David B. Steib, Ph.D., Clinical Psychologist. Also, go to www.cchr.com to educate yourself, for your very life or the life of a love one is at stake as antidepressants are known to cause thoughts of suicide.

Dr. Sunshine

A new study shows that the brain produces more of the mood-lifting chemical serotonin on sunny days than on darker days. https://www.webmd.com/mental-health/news/... /unraveling-suns-role-in-depression.

Earth is a solar-powered world with 98 percent of its warmth coming from sunshine (the rest from geothermal heat). Solar energy lifts rain clouds, drives winds, and sparks the photosynthesis in plants, which feed all living things. A miracle factory is at work just beneath your skin, and when the ultraviolet rays of the sun touch the skin, the factory gets to work. It is a most marvelous system, and without it, you could not remain alive an hour. There are millions of red corpuscles constantly flowing through very small blood vessels throughout every part of the 3,000 square inches of your skin. And there are also tiny oil glands just beneath the skin which biochemists call sterols. As sunshine strikes them, substances within them, called ergo sterols, are irradiated and transformed into vitamin D. Carried to all parts of the body, it enables you to have strong bones, teeth, nails, and a major benefit for the heart.

Every living thing in the world is dependent upon the sun. Without sunshine, nothing could live. In 1877, two researchers, Blunt and Downes, discovered that sunlight can destroy harmful bacteria. Today, it is used to treat bacterial infections. Sunlight on the body dramatically lowers high blood pressure, decreases blood cholesterol, lowers excessively high blood sugars, and increases white blood cells. Adequate sunlight on your body will lower your respiratory rate and will cause your breathing to be slower, deeper, and even easier. Your resting heart rate will decrease, and after exercise it will return to normal much more quickly. Sunlight increases the capacity of the blood to carry oxygen and take it to your body tissues. Even a single exposure to the ultraviolet light in sunlight will greatly increase the oxygen content of your blood, and this effect will continue for several days. Bronchial asthma patients, who could hardly breathe, were able to inhale freely after a sunbath. It is of interest that many of these beneficial effects of sunlight are heightened if a person combines sunbathing with a regular program of physical exercise. Sunlight also stimulate the penial

Dr. Exercise

In numerous studies exercise has been shown to increase both serotonin production and release; In particular, aerobic exercises like running, swimming and biking, are the most likely to boost serotonin. "A 90 minute walk increases serotonin production by 100 percent".

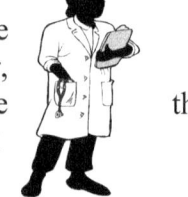

--https://www.psychologytoday.com/blog/prefrontal.../boosting-your-serotonin-activity.

To have optimal health, you have to have perfect circulation of the circulatory system, so oxygen, water, and nutrition can reach every organ of the body, especially the vital organs, i.e. the brain, liver, colon, heart, etc. "You'd have to go a long way to find something as good as exercise as a fountain of youth. And you don't have to run marathons to reap the benefits. Little more than rapid walking for 30 minutes at a time, three or four times a week can provide ten years of rejuvenation" Dr. Roy J. Shepard, University of Toronto. Take a look at the facts. The adage "Use it or lose it" applies not only to muscles and bones but also to hearts, lungs, brains, blood vessels, joints and every other part of the body. A sedentary lifestyle is a direct route to an early grave. Inactivity kills us — literally! A strong genetic inheritance helps some people survive incredible odds. But just living longer isn't today's only concern. Today's concern also includes quality of life and the energy, strength, and health to go with it. I have shared with each of my children, that as I played games like tag, hide-and-seek, and capture-the-flag with them, it is my goal to do the same with my grandchildren.

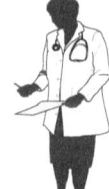

Dr. Water

Neurosci Behav Physiol. 2001 May-Jun;31(3):327-32.

Brain serotonin metabolism during water deprivation and hydration in rats.

Popova NK[1], Ivanova LN, Amstislavskaya TG, Melidi NN, Naumenko KS, Maslova LN, Bulygina VV.

Abstract

The effects of two-day water deprivation and hyperhydration (provision of 4% sucrose solution for 48h) on levels of serotonin and its major metabolite 5-hydroxyindoleacetic acid (5-HIAA) in the midbrain and hypothalamus were studied in Wistar rats. The rates of diuresis (0.05 +/- 0.01 and 0.84 +/- 0.12 ml/h/100 g in water deprivation and hyperhydration respectively) and urine osmolality (1896 +/- 182 and 50 +/- 13 mOsm/kg) reflected increases and decreases in blood vasopressin levels. Water deprivation was associated with a significant increase in 5-HIAA levels in the midbrain and hypothalamus, along with a decrease in serotonin levels and a three-fold increase in serotonin catabolism (the 5-HIAA:serotonin concentration ratio). Hyperhydration induced moderate increases in serotonin and 5-HIAA levels in the hypothalamus with no changes in the midbrain. The blood corticosterone level doubled in water deprivation and decreased in hyperhydration. It is suggested that activation of the serotoninergic system induces a complex adaptive reaction in water deprivation, including mechanisms specific for the regulation of water-electrolyte homeostasis and non-specific stress mechanisms (vasopressin and corticoliberin secretion).

--https://www.ncbi.nlm.nih.gov/pubmed/11430579.
The human adult is made up of approximately 70-80% water. The human brain is about 85% water and a baby is approximately 75% water. The human body is about 80 percent water. So why is this colorless, tasteless, calorie-and-salt-free substance so absolutely necessary? The answer lies in the physiology of the body. It is the lubricant that makes everything else work. It is the water that transports the prescription
drug, herb, vitamin, etc. throughout the body to be where it is needed.
A drink of water is exactly what the body needs to carry out all its life processes. Water is an essential nutrient that is involved in every function of the body. It helps transport nutrients and waste products in and out of cells. It is necessary for all digestive, absorption, circulatory, and excretory functions, as well as for the utilization of the water-soluble vitamins. It is also needed for the maintenance of proper body temperature. By drinking an adequate amount of water each day-50% of your body weight in ounces minimum-you can ensure that your body has a key nutrient it needs to maintain good health.

Drink enough water a day to keep the urine pale. Our kidneys alone process approximately 50 gallons of fluid in a day. In a 24-hour period, more than 8 quarts of digestive juices flow into the digestive tract. Much of this water is recycled over and over again by your kidneys. But about 4 to 6 cups of water a day are lost through the urine, lungs, skin, feces, and perspiration. For this reason, if you do not keep drinking water, your kidneys cannot perform their function well, and this is one reason for kidney disease.
"When we come to the individual need for water, it is readily realized that water is certainly our most precious mineral. It is the most essential of all minerals for our bodies. An animal can lose all its fat, about half its

protein,-but if it loses as much as one-tenth of its water, it will die."- Jonathan Forman, M.D. "Water and Man."

The countless millions of cells inside of you are constantly being bathed in water. And this is not merely a soaking process, but a re-washing activity done by your blood stream. Water in the blood brings nutrition and oxygen to your tissues, and carries off wastes.

All told, a wealth of information has been published on the subject of blood flow characteristics and its impact on a variety of disease states. The research often is published under the title of "hemorheology." This term comes from "hemo" which refers to blood and "rheology" which refers to the study of the flow properties of complex materials. Among the implications of this research is that adequate water drinking combined with other aspects of a healthful lifestyle may help postpone or prevent a variety of diseases and their complications. A few of the benefits that may accrue from improvement in the blood flow caused by a more liberal intake of water are: diabetic complications, stroke, high blood pressure, heart disease, and symptoms of intermittent claudication (leg pain due to blockage in leg
blood vessels).

Many times, people are suffering from lower back pain when most of the time it is their kidneys screaming for more water. The next time you have mild lower back pain try drinking more water and see what happens. Remember there are times when your body requires more water than usual. For example on hot days, during physical exercise, if you have diarrhea or a fever, etc. Toxicity is a major cause of immune system weakening leading to hundreds of diseases, which could be simply eliminated by drinking water. Get into the habit of drinking water liberally. To systematically hydrate the body, one should drink four ounces of water every waking hour. Drink on arising, having one to two glasses of water before breakfast, in midmorning and mid-afternoon. Start the day off right. Give the early morning drink some zest by adding a twist of lemon. Real natural lemon and your liver were made for each other. Try replacing the coffee stimulation with a glass of water and quality vitamins; also avoid the nervous system disorders caused by caffeine. When tempted to snack between meals weakening your digestive system, reach for a glass of water and drink liberally, habitual hunger pangs will soon go away. I highly recommend the book "Your Body's Many Cries For Water" by F. Batmanghelidg, M.D. or go to www.watercure.com.

Dr. Fresh Air

80% of human energy comes from the atmosphere. It is more than just Nitrogen and Oxygen that the boy takes from the air. A vast amount of trace minerals exist in the atmosphere due to the cleansing action of the oceans of the world. These are in parts per billion and smaller.

"The lungs are constantly throwing off impurities, and they need to be constantly supplied with fresh air." The Ministry of Healing, Pacific Press Publishing Association, Ellen White, p. 274.

Throughout most of recorded history, it seems that people have taken fresh air for granted. However, with the advent of the industrial revolution, followed by current concerns for indoor and outdoor air pollution, fresh air has become a more valued commodity. Air is composed of about 20 percent oxygen. It takes approximately 9 percent to sustain human life, presently there are major U.S. cities whose oxygen content is down to 12 percent. Fresh air is chemically different than the re-circulated indoor air that most people breathe. High quality fresh air is actually electrified. The life-giving oxygen molecule is negatively charged or "negatively ionized." This negatively charged oxygen gives rise to a number of benefits; improved sense of well-being, increased rate and quality of growth in plants and animals, improved function of the lung's protective cilia, tranquilization and relaxation (decreased anxiety), lowered body temperature, lowered resting heart rate, decreased survival of bacteria and viruses in the air, improved learning in mammals, and decreased severity of stomach ulcers.

"In order to have good blood, we must breathe well. Full, deep inspirations of pure air, which fill the lungs with oxygen, and purify the blood is crucial. They impart to it a bright color and send it-a life-giving current-to every part of the body. A good respiration soothes the nerves; it stimulates the appetite and renders digestion more perfect; and it induces sound, refreshing sleep. If an insufficient supply of oxygen is received, the blood moves sluggishly. The waste, poisonous matter, which should be thrown off in the exhalations from the lungs, is retained, and the blood becomes impure. Not only the lungs, but the stomach, liver, and brain are affected. The skin becomes sallow, digestion is retarded; the heart is depressed; the brain clouded; the thoughts are confused; gloom settles upon the spirits; the whole system becomes [depressed] and inactive, and peculiarly susceptible to disease." Ellen White, The Ministry of Healing, p. 272-273.

Along with improper breathing techniques, "many health professionals also believe the current rise in breathing problems is linked to pollution. We tend to think of breathing as simply taking in air. But that's just the first step. Your lungs also need to be able to absorb the oxygen out of the air you inhale. Then you must be able to expel the carbon dioxide from your lungs to make way for the next batch of air. When any of these steps break down, breathing troubles begin. You will cough, choke, wheeze and gasp; develop asthma, bronchitis and emphysema; and eventually die. When your lungs are not functioning at their peak capacity and it's hard to breathe, you can neither expel carbon dioxide nor deliver the optimal amount of oxygen to your body. This can cause your body to shut down." Journal of Longevity, vol. 9/No 7, p. 3, 5.

"Fresh air will prove far more beneficial to sick persons than medicine, and is far more essential to them than their food… Thousands have died for want of pure water and pure air, which might have lived." White, Counsels on Health, p. 55.

The human body operates on oxygen. Make sure your get enough by exercising, keeping your house well ventilated even in winter, and pausing frequently to take slow deep breaths. Place one hand on your chest and the other on your stomach. Breathe normally for a few moments, noting the movement of each hand as you inhale. Which hand rises more dramatically? If it is the one on your belly, take it off and pat yourself on the back. You have excellent respiration technique. But if it's the hand on your chest, you'd better take a deep breath—though you probably can't. You're breathing wrong. To breathe properly try this simple breathing exercise. It will energize and refresh you. Stand or sit with your back straight. Exhale deeply through your mouth. Now, draw the air back into your lungs. As you do, imagine it going right down into your belly, filling it. Feel your stomach expand as you inhale. When your lungs are full, slowly begin to exhale. It should take you a little bit longer to exhale than it does to inhale. Tighten the muscles of your stomach as you gently push the last bit of air out. Repeat the process, slowly, five or six times, several times a day. The fresh morning air is best, if possible step outdoors into the fresh air. You can also flush your body with oxygen by exercising. Activity opens up blood vessels and speeds those oxygen-laden red blood cells on their rounds. And remember the house plants. Placing at least one plant for every 100 square feet of indoor space is recommended. Live plants not only eat many toxic pollutants and freshen the air with oxygen; they probably slip in some extra negative ions as well. Remember a meal eaten of high-fat reduces your blood's ability to carry oxygen. I highly recommend you read the book entitled Why is Fresh Air Fresh? By Dr. Bernell Baldwin.

Dr. Rest

In recent years, melatonin, a natural body hormone, has been found to enhance sleep. Melatonin levels reach a peak in children, then falls slowly and steadily throughout adult life. This may explain why children sleep so much better than older people. The body carefully regulates melatonin production. The process is largely controlled by the light-dark cycle. Optimal melatonin production occurs only at night, in a dark environment.

The pineal gland, located in the center of the brain, is the "clock" that regulates this process at the right time. Melatonin is not stored in the body. We need a liberal supply each evening to sleep well. Studies demonstrate that daily exposure to natural sunlight will boost melatonin output. Artificial light is a weak substitute, as well as manufactured supplements.

Rest is what the human family needs; physical rest, mental rest, and spiritual rest. "The stomach, when we lie down to rest, should have its work all done, that it may enjoy rest, as well as other portions of the body. The work of digestion should not be carried on through any period of the sleeping hours. After the stomach, which has been overtaxed, has performed its task, it becomes exhausted, which causes faintness. Here many are deceived, and think that it is the want of food which produces such feelings, and without giving the stomach time to rest, they take more food, which for the time removes the faintness. And the more the appetite is indulged, the more will be its clamors for gratification. This faintness is generally the result of meat eating, and eating frequently, and too much. The stomach becomes weary by being kept constantly at work, disposing of food not the most healthful. Having no time for rest, the digestive organs become enfeebled, hence the sense of "goneness," and desire for frequent eating. The remedy such require, is to eat less frequently and less liberally, and be satisfied with plain, simple food, eating twice, or, at most, three times a day. The stomach must have its regular periods for labor and rest; hence eating irregularly and between meals, is a most pernicious violation of the laws of health. With regular habits, and proper food, the stomach will gradually recover." Ellen White, Counsels on Diet and Foods, pg. 175.

Just as the body has a natural daily clock called circadian rhythm, it also has a weekly clock called circaseptan rhythm. Circaseptan rhythms are just that: body rhythms that run about seven days in length. Medical research has demonstrated such rhythms in connection with a variety of physiological functions. Some that have been identified include heart rate, suicides, natural hormones in human breast milk, swelling after surgery, and rejection of transplanted organs. Many cultures have experimented with a weekly cycle, including France during the French Revolution, going to a 7-day work week with disastrous results. Others have pointed to an even more compelling reason for the existence of the weekly cycle: it is the way God created us. Indeed, in the book of Genesis, the seven-day weekly cycle is described as part of God's design in creation. You can take one day in seven and rest for physical health, but the seventh day Sabbath is required for spiritual health. "Let us labor therefore to enter into that rest, lest any man fall after the same example of unbelief." Hebrews 4:11.

"The restfulness which is in Christ Jesus, the peace of Christ, how precious, how healing its influence, how soothing to the oppressed soul! However dark his prospects, let him cherish a spirit to hope for good. While nothing is gained by despondency, much is lost. While cheerfulness and a calm resignation and peace will make others happy and healthy, it will be of the greatest benefit to oneself. Sadness and talking of disagreeable things is encouraging the disagreeable scenes, bringing back upon oneself the disagreeable effect. God wants us to forget all these—not look down but up, up!"

Ellen White, Mind, Character, and Personality Volume 2, pg. 662.

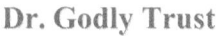

Dr. Godly Trust

When a person is struggling with depression, especially the youth, religion or better yet a personal relationship with God the Father and His son Jesus Christ play an important role in rebalancing the mind. Notice these five facts:

1. Suicide rates had a negative correlation with religiosity.
2. Church attendance was a major predictor in suicide, even more then employment.
3. There is a negative correlation between drug use and religiousness.
4. Church attendance was found to be more of an indicator of drug abstinence than parents.
5. Use of alcohol: Most research finding support that religious affiliation, especially participation, lowers the rate of alcohol consumption.

Bailey CM. The effects of religion on mental health: Implications for Seventh-day Adventist. 20th International Faith and Learning Seminar held at Loma Linda University, Loma Linda California, USA June 15-26, 1997.

[A Psalm] of David. *"Bless the LORD, O my soul: and all that is within me, [bless] his holy name. Bless the LORD, O my soul, and forget not all His benefits: Who forgiveth all thine iniquities; who healeth all thy diseases*;" Psalms 103:1-3.

Christian meditation and prayer have their greatest benefits when they provide a respite from stressful thoughts and feelings, and an opportunity to find solutions for dealing with life's most pressing stressors. For such processes to occur, the reasoning powers of the brain must be active during the meditative process. Our high intellectual powers, including spiritual reasoning, reside in the part of the brain called the frontal lobe. When this brain region is intimately involved in our thinking, a type of brain wave called the beta wave predominates. If you were to measure brain activity with an electroencephalogram (EEG) and it shows the beta wave, it would indicate that healthy thinking is occurring, characterized by dynamic frontal lobe activity.

Studies show that Christian meditation involves the frontal lobe and beta activity. This is what one would expect. After all, prayer from the Bible perspective is an extremely active process. Whether we are reflecting on God's goodness, thanking Him for helping us in specific ways, seeking to know His will in a perplexing situation, or praying for individuals who have specific needs, Christian meditation and prayer involve an active frontal lobe.

In the medical literature, there are indications those individuals who trust God live longer. For example, Dr. Jeremy Kark and colleagues recently compared two ethnically Jewish groups that seemed to be very similar except for religious observance.

Among members of a secular community, the risk of death at any age was nearly doubled that of those members of a religious community, that is, those who were religiously observant. (Kark JD, Shemi G, et al. Does religious observance promote health? <u>Mortality in secular vs religious kibbutzim in Israel</u>. *Am J Public Health* 1996 Mar; 86(3):341-346.

- In a similar study, recent stressful life events increased the risk of health problems in a secular community. Members of a comparative religious community seemed to be protected from the negative effects of stress. Dr. Kark's team proposed some reasons why the members of the religious community experienced stress-buffering and improved longevity: Emotional well–being fostered by a sense of belonging to a religious community.
- Belief in God.
- A relaxation response induced by frequent prayer.
- Highly stable marital and family bonding.

➢ Social support providing a buffer against stressful life events.

One fascinating study looked at the religious experience of those Americans who reached the golden age of 100. Among the centenarians, the researchers found that religiosity significantly enhanced physical health. Although there are still many unanswered questions, the benefits of trust in God are due to more than simply attending religious services. (Levin JS, Vanderpool HY. Is frequent religious attendance really conducive to better health? Towards an epidemiology of religion. Soc Sci Med 1987;24(7):589-600.)

Furthermore, the far-reaching benefits of faith seem to transcend age and racial boundaries. A study of African-Americans found that those who engage in organized religious activities had improved health and life satisfaction. (Levin JS, Chatters LM, Taylor RJ. Religious effects on health status and life satisfaction among African Americans. J Gerontol B Psychol Sci Soc 1995 May; 50 (3): S154-163.)

Even those who engage in religious pursuits outside of organizational structure experienced this boost in satisfaction. Indeed, one of the most consistent findings-across racial groups-is that spirituality profoundly improves quality of life. The profound benefits in the quality of life brought about by exercising faith are described by a Duke University researcher who stated:

➢ Religious attendance and private devotion strengthen a person's religious belief system.
➢ Strong religious belief systems, in turn, when accompanied by a high level of religious certainty, have a substantial positive influence on well-being.
➢ Individual with strong religious faith report:
✓ Higher levels of life satisfaction
✓ Greater personal happiness
✓ Fewer negative psychosocial consequences of traumatic life events

Ellison CG. Religious involvement and subjective well-being. J Health Soc Behav 1991 Mar;32(1):80-99. Proof Positive, Neil Nedly, M.D. p. 506.

Religious people are happier, study finds
▸ People who follow a religion through active participation in congregations tend to be happier, according to a new study.
▸ The study by Pew Research Centre, a nonpartisan fact tank, compared the lives of religious people and non-religious people by analyzing survey data from more than two dozen countries including the United States, Mexico, and Australia.

--Chelsea Ritschel 6 Feb. 2019 https://www.msn.com

Where do you turn for renewal? What is at your core, your center of being? Take some time to step back and think about what is truly important to you. Look beyond the clamor of daily activity to the universal themes of life. Choose an inspiring book, listen to some uplifting music, give thanks for the marvelous gift of life and health. Every breath you take is a miracle. Every morning is the beginning of the rest of your life; a gift from God. Religion then, is not a piece of information for the mind. It is a way of life, which includes all that we are, all that we do all our hope and aspirations, all the moments of our lives.

Chapter IV: True and false Systems of Mind Cure

"The sympathy which exists between the mind and the body is very great. When one is affected, the other responds. The condition of the mind has much to do with the health of the physical system. If the mind is free and happy under a consciousness of right doing and a sense of satisfaction in causing happiness to others, it will create a cheerfulness that will react upon the whole system, causing a freer circulation of the blood and a toning up of the entire body. The blessing of God is a healer; and those who are abundant in benefiting others will realize that wondrous blessing in their hearts and lives". White, Medical Ministry (M.M.), p. 105.1.

Thousands Needlessly Sick

"Thousands are sick and dying around us who might get well and live if they would; but their imagination holds them. They fear that they will be made worse if they labor or exercise, when this is just the change they need to make them well. Without this they never can improve. They should exercise the power of the will, rise above their aches and debility, engage in useful employment, and forget that they have aching backs, sides, lungs, and heads. Neglecting to exercise the entire body, or a portion of it, will bring on morbid conditions. Inaction of any of the organs of the body will be followed by a decrease in size and strength of the muscles, and will cause the blood to flow sluggishly through the blood vessels". White, M.M. p. 105.2.

Health through Service for Others

"Those who, so far as it is possible, engage in the work of doing good to others by giving practical demonstration of their interest in them, are not only relieving the ills of human life in helping them bear their burdens, but are at the same time contributing largely to their own health of soul and body. Doing good is a work that benefits both giver and receiver. If you forget self in your interest for others, you gain a victory over your infirmities. The satisfaction you will realize in doing good will aid you greatly in the recovery of the healthy tone of the imagination.

The pleasure of doing good animates the mind and vibrates through the whole body. While the faces of benevolent men are lighted up with cheerfulness, and their countenances express the moral elevation of the mind, those of selfish, stingy men are dejected, cast down, and gloomy. Their moral defects are seen in their countenances....

Invalids, I advise you to venture something. Arouse your willpower, and at least make a trial of this matter. Withdraw your thoughts and affections from yourselves. Walk out by faith. Are you inclined to center your thoughts upon yourselves, fearing to exercise, and fearing that if you expose yourself to the air you will lose your life; resist these thoughts and feelings. Do not yield to your diseased imagination". White, MM, p. 105.3.

Drudgery versus Healthful Activity
Manual labor quickens the circulation of the blood. The more active the circulation the more free will be the blood from obstructions and impurities. The blood nourishes the body. The health of the body depends upon the healthful circulation of the blood. If work is performed without the heart being in it, it is simply drudgery, and the benefit which should result from the exercise is not gained. White, MM, p. 106.3.

Contentment and Cheerfulness
A contented mind, a cheerful spirit, is health to the body and strength to the soul. Nothing is so fruitful a cause of disease as depression, gloominess, and sadness. Mental depression is terrible. White, MM, p.106.4.

Enlisting the Willpower
"*In journeying I have met many who were really sufferers through their imaginations. They lacked willpower to rise above and combat disease of body and mind, and therefore they were held in suffering bondage. A large share of this class of invalids is found among the youth. I sometimes meet with young women lying in bed sick. They complain of headache. Their pulse may be firm, and they be full in flesh; yet their sallow skins indicate that they are bilious. My thoughts have been that, if I were in their condition, I should know at once what course to pursue to obtain relief. Although I might feel indisposed, I should not expect to recover while lying in bed. I should bring willpower to my aid, and should leave my bed and engage in active physical exercise. I should strictly observe regular habits of rising early. I should eat sparingly, thus relieving my system of unnecessary burden, and should encourage cheerfulness, and give myself the benefits of proper exercise in the open air. I should bathe frequently, and drink freely of pure, soft water. If this course should be*

followed perseveringly, resisting the inclination to do otherwise, it would work wonders in the recovery of health". White, MM, p. 106.5.

Deceptive Ailments

"I feel sad for those who are not only deceived themselves in thinking that they are sick, but who are kept deceived by their parents and friends, who pet their ailments and relieve them from labor. If these were so situated as to be compelled to labor, they would scarcely notice difficulties which, while indolent, keep them in bed. Physical exercise is a precious blessing for both mental and physical ailments. Exercise, with cheerfulness, would in many cases prove a most effective restorer to the complaining invalid. Useful employment would bring into exercise the enfeebled muscles, and would enliven the stagnant blood in the system, and would arouse the torpid liver to perform its work. The circulation of the blood would be equalized and the entire system invigorated to overcome bad conditions. I frequently turn from the bedside of these self-made invalids, saying to myself, Dying by inches, dying of indolence, a disease which no one but themselves can cure. I sometimes see young men and women who might be a blessing to their parents, if they would share with them the cares and burdens of life. But they feel no disposition to do this, because it is not agreeable but is attended with some weariness. They devote much of their time in vain amusement, to the neglect of duties necessary for them to perform in order to obtain an experience which will be of great value to them in their future battles with the difficulties of real life. They live for the present only, and neglect the physical, mental, and moral qualifications which would fit them for the emergencies of life and give them self-reliance and self-respect in times of trial and of danger". White, MM, p. 107.1.

The Holy Spirit as a Restorative

"Many doctors have made a great mistake in regard to exercise and amusements, and a still greater in their teaching concerning religious experience and religious excitement. The religion of the Bible is not detrimental to the health of body or mind. The exalting influence of the Spirit of God is the best restorative for the sick. Heaven is all health, and the more fully the heavenly influences are felt, the more sure the recovery of the believing invalid...."""Let invalids do something, instead of occupying their minds with a simple play, which lowers them in their own estimation and leads them to think their lives useless. Keep the power of the will awake, for the will aroused and rightly directed is a potent soother of the nerves. Invalids are far happier to be employed, and their recovery is more easily affected". White, MM, p. 108.1.

Sanctified Mind Cure
The light given me is that if the sister you mention would brace up and cultivate her taste for wholesome food, all these sinking spells would pass away. She has cultivated her imagination; the enemy has taken advantage of her weakness of body, and her mind is not braced to bear up against the hardships of everyday life. It is good, sanctified mind cure she needs, an increase of faith, and active service for Christ. She needs also the exercise of her muscles in outside practical labor. Physical exercise will be to her one of the greatest blessings of her life. She need not be an invalid, but a wholesome-minded, healthy woman, prepared to act her part nobly and well. All the treatment that may be given to this sister will be of little advantage unless she acts her part. She needs to strengthen muscle and nerve by physical labor. She need not be an invalid, but can do good, earnest labor. Like many others, she has a diseased imagination. But she can overcome and be a healthy woman. I have had this message to give too many, and with the best results."White, MM, p. 108.3.

Chronic Invalidism
"Once I was called to see a young woman with whom I was well acquainted. She was sick, and was running down fast. Her mother wished me to pray for her. The mother stood there weeping and saying, "Poor child; she cannot live long." I felt her pulse. I prayed with her, and then addressed her, "My sister, if you get up and dress and go to your usual work in the office, all this invalidism will pass away." "Do you think this would pass away?" she said. "Certainly," I said. "You have nearly smothered the life forces by invalidism." I turned to the mother and told her that her daughter would have died of a diseased imagination if they had not been convinced of their error. She had been educating herself to invalidism. Now this is a very poor school. But I said to her, "Change this order; arise and dress." She was obedient, and is alive today". White, MM, p. 109.1.

"Exercise will aid the work of digestion. To walk out after a meal, hold the head erect, put back the shoulders, and exercise moderately, will be a great benefit. The mind will be diverted from self to the beauties of nature. The less the attention is called to the stomach after a meal, the better. If you are in constant fear that your food will hurt you, it most assuredly will. Forget self, and think of something cheerful". White, MM, p. 109.2.

Inspire the Despondent
"Tell the suffering ones of a compassionate Saviour.... He looks with compassion upon those who regard their case as hopeless. While the soul

is filled with fear and terror, the mind cannot see the tender compassion of Christ. Our sanitariums are to be an agency for bringing peace and rest to the troubled minds. If you can inspire the despondent with hopeful, saving faith, contentment and cheerfulness will take the place of discouragement and unrest. Wonderful changes can then be wrought in their physical condition. Christ will restore both body and soul, and, realizing His compassion and love, they will rest in Him. He is the bright and morning Star, shining amid the moral darkness of this sinful, corrupt world. He is the Light of the world, and all who give their hearts to Him will find peace, rest, and joy". White, MM, p. 109.3.

Counterfeit Miracles

"Satan is a diligent Bible student. He knows that his time is short, and he seeks at every point to counterwork the work of the Lord upon this earth. It is impossible to give any idea of the experience of the people of God who shall be alive upon the earth when celestial glory and a repetition of the persecutions of the past are blended. They will walk in the light proceeding from the throne of God. By means of the angels there will be constant communication between heaven and earth. And Satan, surrounded by evil angels and claiming to be God, will work miracles of all kinds, to deceive, if possible, the very elect. God's people will not find their safety in working miracles; for Satan will counterfeit the miracles that will be wrought. God's tried and tested people will find their power in the sign spoken of in Exodus 31:12-18. They are to take their stand on the living word, "It is written." This is the only foundation upon which they can stand securely. Those who have broken their covenant with God will in that day be without God and without hope".—Testimonies for the Church vol.9, p. 16.1.

Taking Hold of the Eternal

"The mind cure must be free from all human enchantment. It must not grovel to humanity but soar aloft to the spiritual, taking hold of the eternal". White, MM, p. 110.3

Satan's Apparent Miracles

"We are to be on guard against Satan's deceptive arts. He will take possession of human bodies, and make men and women sick. Then he will suddenly cease to exercise his evil power, and it will be proclaimed that a miracle has been wrought. We need now to have a true understanding of the power of Jesus Christ to save to the uttermost all who come unto Him.... Men and women are not to study the science of how to take captive the minds of those who associate with them. This is the science that Satan teaches. We are to resist everything of the kind. We are not to tamper with mesmerism and hypnotism— the science of the one who lost his first estate and was cast out of the heavenly courts. The science of a pure, wholesome, consistent Christian life is obtained by studying the word of the Lord. This is the highest education that any earthly being can obtain. These are the lessons that the students in our schools are to be taught, that they may come forth with pure thoughts and clean minds and hearts, prepared to ascend the ladder of progress and to practice the Christian virtues". White, MM, p. 110.4

Efforts of Satan to Confuse Minds

"For thousands of years Satan has been experimenting upon the properties of the human mind, and he has learned to know it well. By his subtle workings in these last days he is linking the human mind with his own, imbuing it with his thoughts; and he is doing this work in so deceptive a manner that those who accept his guidance know not that they are being led by him at his will. The great deceiver hopes so to confuse the minds of men and women that none but his voice will be heard". White, MM, p. 111.2

A Dangerous System of Mind Cure

"I am so weighed down in your case that I must continue to write to you, lest in your blindness you will not see where you need to reform. I am instructed that you are entertaining ideas with which God has forbidden you to deal. I will name these as a species of mind cure. You suppose that you can use this mind cure in your professional work as a physician. In tones of earnest warning the words were spoken: Beware, beware where your feet are placed and your mind is carried. God has not appointed you this work. The theory of mind controlling mind is originated by Satan to introduce himself as the chief worker, to put human philosophy where divine philosophy should be. No man or woman should exercise his or her will to control the senses or reason of another, so that the mind of the person is rendered passively subject to the will of the one who is exercising the control. This science may appear to be something beautiful, but it is a science which you are in no case to handle.... There is something better for you to engage in than the control of human nature over human nature. I lift the danger signal. The only safe and true mind cure covers much. The physician must educate the people to look from the human to the divine. He who has made man's mind knows precisely what the mind needs. In taking up the science you have begun to advocate, you are giving an education which is not safe for you or for those you teach. It is dangerous to tinge minds with the science of mind cure". White, MM, p. 111.3.

A Deceptive Fallacy

"This science may appear to you to be very valuable; but to you and to *others it is a fallacy prepared by Satan. It is the charm of the serpent which stings to spiritual death. It covers much that seems wonderful, but it is foreign to the nature and spirit of Christ. This science does not lead to Him who is life and salvation. The poor, afflicted souls with whom you are brought in contact have needed more of your attention than they have received. You have it in your power to encourage them to look to Jesus, and, by beholding, be changed to His image. The true knowledge of Jesus Christ will lead your mind ... in a safe direction. It gives the inspiration of true worship. It is the fellowship of the soul with Him who is its life. Coming in contact with Him, the mind is drawn to His heart of life and is inspired with the essence of His sanctification. Be careful, my brother, ... in regard to where your faith is tending. Jesus lives to make intercession for you. Let your mind be one with the mind of Christ. Having His mind, you will not soar to heights which will at last bring you down to the lowest depths. Dabble not in those things which now appear to you so attractive, but which do not lead to Christ. Let your ambition ascend higher, to pure, true fellowship with Him in whom you may safely glory. Then your religion will be a power for good. You will not then communicate that which will prove a snare unto death." White, MM, p. 112.3.*

A Call to Perfection

"Our Saviour understood all about human nature, and He says to every human being, "Be ye therefore perfect, even as your Father which is in heaven is perfect." As God is perfect in His sphere, so man is to be perfect in his sphere. Those who receive Christ are among the number to whom the words so full of hope are spoken, "As many as received Him, to them gave He power to become the sons of God, even to them that believe on His name." These words declare to us that we should be content with nothing less than the best and highest character, a character formed after the divine similitude. When such a character is possessed, the life, the faith, the purity of the religion, is an instructive example to others. "Righteousness exalteth a nation: but sin is a reproach to any people..." "I fear, lest by any means, as the serpent beguiled Eve through his subtlety, so your minds should be corrupted from the simplicity that is in Christ." ... "Put on the whole armor of God that ye may be able to stand against the wiles of the devil. For we wrestle not against flesh and blood, but against principalities, against powers, against the rulers of the darkness of this world, against spiritual wickedness in high places. Wherefore take unto you the whole armor of Go that ye may be able to withstand in the evil day, and having done all, to stand. Stand therefore, having your loins girt about with truth, and having on the breastplate of

righteousness; and your feet shod with the preparation of the gospel of peace; above all, taking the shield of faith, wherewith ye shall be able to quench all the fiery darts of the wicked. And take the helmet of salvation, and the sword of the Spirit, which is the word of God." White, MM, p. 112.7.

Personal Experience in Meeting False Science
"At the beginning of my work I had the mind-cure science to contend with. I was sent from place to place to declare the falseness of this science, into which many were entering. The mind cure was entered upon very innocently—to relieve the tension upon the minds of nervous invalids. But, oh, how sad were the results! God sent me from place to place to rebuke everything pertaining to this science. I wish to speak plainly to you. You have entered upon a work which has no place in the work of a Christian physician, and which must find no place in our health institutions. Innocent though it may appear, this mind cure, if exercised upon the patients, will in its development be for their destruction, not their restoration. The third chapter of Second Timothy describes persons who accept error, such as one mind exercising complete control over another mind. God forbids any such thing. The mind cure is one of Satan's greatest sciences, and it is important that our physicians see clearly the real character of this science; for through it great temptations will come to them. This science must not be allowed a particle of standing room in our sanitariums." White, MM, p. 113.3.

Through the Mind Satan May Control the Body
"God has not given one ray of light or encouragement for our physicians to take up the work of having one mind completely control the mind of another, so that one acts out the will of another. Let us learn the ways and purposes of God. Let not the enemy gain the least advantage over you. Let him not lead you to dare to endeavor to control another mind until it becomes a machine in your hands. This is the science of Satan's working. Thus he works when he entices men to sell the soul for liquor. He takes possession of body, mind, and soul, and it is no longer the man, but Satan, who acts. And the cruelty of Satan is expressed as the drunkard lifts his hand to strike down the wife he has promised to love and cherish as long as life shall last. The deeds of the drunkard are an expression of Satan's violence". White, MM, p. 114.1.

A Positive Peril
"Now, my brother, I consider you to be in positive peril. I present this because I know that you are in great danger of being seduced by Satan. We are living in a time when every phase of fanaticism will press its way in among believers and unbelievers. Satan will come in, speaking lies in

hypocrisy. Everything that he can invent to deceive men and women will be brought forward. Just in proportion as men lose their sense of the need of vital religion, so they become filled with common, earthly ideas, which they exalt as wonderful knowledge. Physicians who lose their hold on Christ become filled with ideas of their own, which they look upon as some wonderful science, to be brought into the medical profession as something new and strange. I have been awakened at the early hour of twelve to write out these things. Let me tell you plainly that you are in an uncertain condition of mind, and that the efforts you put forth to rescue yourself are in vain. No man can serve two masters. If you try to serve the world and the Lord at the same time, the result will be that worldly policy and worldly schemes will become supreme in your life. Why? Because the word of God will become uncongenial; for the heart is not committed to the molding and fashioning of the Holy Spirit. The will is not given up to God, and therefore enmity to God is revealed. The natural impulses of the heart, ministering to the natural man, are chosen to control.... My brother, while you cherish your own suppositions as truth, God cannot enlighten you. With your present phase of character, you are not capable of understanding the best course to pursue in introducing principles which rest upon a solid basis. Your greatest consideration is, "Is my proper position recognized? Am I called upon as I should be to decide matters?" Your selfish ideas must never become the ruling power in any sanitarium. You are to blend with other men and women who have understanding...Our physicians must not rest content with a half conversion. They need to place their whole trust in Christ. Then the healthy beats of a new heart will change the atmosphere surrounding the soul. Make sure that you are accepted by Christ because you rely on the merits of a crucified and risen Saviour. His righteousness must be your righteousness. He wrought it out for you, and when you receive it you stand justified in the presence of God". White, MM, p. 114.2.

Directing the Mind to Christ

"Christ, the Mighty Healer, is to be exalted—and not any human physician. Physicians, Jesus will hear your prayers. Nurses, if you have a living connection with God, you can in confidence present the sick before Him. He will comfort and bless the suffering ones, molding and fashioning the mind, inspiring it with faith and hope and courage. The Christ life, the Christ grace, is the only power that can safely be brought to bear upon the human mind. Every other influence is to be taken away. No individual should be permitted to take control of another person's mind, thinking that in so doing he is causing him to receive great benefit.

The mind cure is one of the most dangerous deceptions which can be practiced upon any individual. Temporary relief may be felt, but the mind of the one thus controlled is never again so strong and reliable. We may be as weak as was the woman who touched the hem of Christ's garment; but if we use our God-given opportunity to come to Him in faith, He will respond as quickly as He did to that touch of faith.

It is not God's design for any human being to yield his mind to another human being. The risen Christ, who is now set down on the throne at the right hand of the Father, is the Mighty Healer. Look to Him for healing power. Through Him alone can sinners come to God just as they are. Never can they come through any man's mind. The human agent must never interpose between the heavenly agencies and those who are suffering. Everyone should be in a position to cooperate with God in directing the minds of others to Him. Tell them of the grace and power of Him who is the greatest Physician the world ever knew. He came to the world to restore in man the moral image of God. Seeing that Satan was exercising a controlling influence over the minds of men and women in order to further his evil designs, Christ came to combat the powers of darkness, to break the control which Satan had gained over human minds. Make the Saviour the center of attraction. A minister once said that he could but think that Christ must have known something about science. Of what could this minister have been thinking? Science! Christ could have opened door after door of science. He could have revealed to men treasures of science on which they might have feasted to the present time. But knowing that this knowledge would have been appropriated to unholy uses, He did not open the door". White, MM, p. 115.3.

A Perilous Science

"We do not ask you to place yourself under the control of any man's mind. The mind cure is the most awful science which has ever been advocated. Every wicked being can use it in carrying through his own evil designs. We have no business with any such science. We should be afraid of it. Never should the first principles of it be brought into any institution. Christ can do nothing for those who are yoked up with the enemy. His invitation to us is, "Come unto Me, all ye that labor and are heavy-laden, and I will give you rest. Take My yoke upon you, and learn of Me; for I am meek and lowly in heart: and ye shall find rest unto your souls. For My yoke is easy, and My burden is light." When in our daily experience we learn His meekness and lowliness, we find rest. There is then no necessity to search for some mysterious science to soothe the sick. We already have the science which gives them real rest—the science of *salvation, the science of restoration, the science of a living faith in a living Saviour'.* White, M.M., p. 116.4.

Mental Needs Are as Important as Physical—*Some parents attend carefully to the temporal wants of their children; they kindly and faithfully nurse them in sickness, and then think their duty done. Here they mistake. Their work has but just begun. The wants of the mind should be cared for. It requires skill to apply the proper remedies to cure a wounded mind".* White, CG, p. 206.3.

Chapter V: Make A New You Physically & Spiritually: John 3:3

"Health is a matter of choice, not a mystery of chance."
-Robert A. Mendelsohn, M.D.

Humans are composed of about 300 trillion cells. Of these cells, there are millions that die each day and are replaced by the one million cells that are born each and every hour of every day. The complexity of the cellular activities may be better understood by the realization that just one liver cell may contain at least 1,000 enzymes (a protein substance) to assist and speed along reactions which will occur at the rate of over 1,000 times per second. The cell is responsible for everything that occurs in the body.

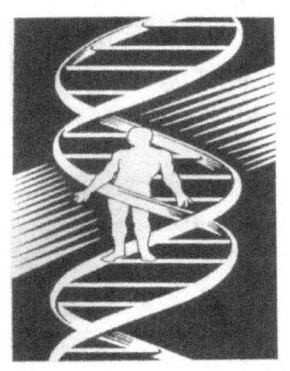

Everything starts at the cellular level, including health and sickness. "If the foundation be destroyed, what can the righteous do"? Psalm 11:3.

The cell has what is known as "cellular intelligence," and has the ability to sample the entire body environment (Inner Terrain) and determine what type of raw materials and fluid are needed and transport them to that site to be utilized. The cells are also sensitive to the consumption of too much refined or processed foods which may upset the potassium/sodium balance, throwing the cell out of balance and making it difficult to control fluids and to clear toxins efficiently.

How to Build a New and Healthy You

Every 90 days the blood cells renew.
Every 3 years the soft tissue renew.
Every 7 years hard tissue renews.
The quality of the new you depend upon:
• The condition of the walls of the small intestines.
• Nutrient bioavailability.
• The quality and the quantity of the food we eat.

- The quality and the type of supplements we take.
- The number of factors that affect our biochemical efficiency.

As you can see, time becomes a very important factor. We must be patient with nature while we continue to do the right things. The X factor makes the difference. At age 20, it takes X amount of minerals to build a cell; at age 40 it takes 2X; age 60 it takes 3X; at age 80 it takes 4X. At age 20 it takes 6 months to restore the body's energy, at age 40 – 12 months; at age 60 – 18 months; at age 80 – 24 months, all things being normal.

Cells do not live forever! They are continually replacing themselves and producing new cells. This means that you are constantly replacing the old worn-out cells with fresh, new cells. The importance of this is quite significant; however, most people rarely think twice about this phenomenon. Your body is actually being reborn piece by piece, or I should say cell by cell. This is true healing, God's way of healing without drugs or side effects.

The cells of the bloodstream are capable of replacing themselves every 90 days. They are some of the hardest working cells of the body and tend to wear out faster than other cells. Their main functions are to carry oxygen to the cells, to carry toxins out of the body, and to fight foreign invaders that take advantage of imbalances in your body chemistry. The cells of the soft tissue are capable of replacing themselves every three years. This means that all your organs, i.e. pancreas, heart, lungs, liver, kidneys, etc, are reborn every three years, depending on the cycle the cells are in. Cells are not replaced all at the same time within the three year cycle; every cell of an organ will have replaced itself.

The cells of the hard tissues are reborn every seven years. These include all your bones. When you give your body the raw material i.e. minerals, follow God's eight natural laws of health, and balance your body chemistry, then the new cells will be healthier than the cells they replace. Eventually, you will regain optimal health and be restored to the image of God. That is why it took a year and three months to heal my pancreas at age 26. James says, "But let patience have [her] perfect work, that ye may be perfect and entire, wanting nothing" James 1:4. It takes time to heal as the above information points out, but we have been programmed to want instant relief at whatever the cost. God says, "My people are destroyed for lack of knowledge: because thou hast rejected knowledge, I will also reject thee, that thou shalt be no priest to me: seeing thou hast forgotten the law of thy God, I will also forget thy children" Hosea 4:6. Christians perish because of a lack of knowledge of anatomy, physiology and God's eight natural laws of health and simple remedies.

As you allow nature to heal you, one day you start to notice symptoms like, itching, tiredness, constipation, etc, will be gone. The disappearance of these symptoms is your evidence that your body is in the healing process and if you are patient and help nature and not hinder her, you will recover health. That is why a little pill, which is void of life itself, which has no nutritional value, and turns your pH acid, cannot and will not ever be able to heal.

Chapter VI: What You Can do to Strengthen Your Will

- Practice deciding things-make up your mind positively, immediately after you have weighted the facts-and stick by your decision, willing to change only when the contrary facts are overwhelming. It is often better to make a mistake, than to sit on the fence of indecision! Sometimes writing the choice or decision down helps a person stick to the decision they make.
- Complete each job before you begin another. Don't flit from one thing to another and from one room to another, traveling in a circle.
- Sometimes games can help develop the ability to decide. I had a young patient who had a reputation among the hospital staff for being excellent at table tennis. But when I played with him, he kept moving back and forth trying to decide when to serve the ball. Once he did, he could really play. Playing that game helped him to make his decision sooner until he could serve with decisiveness.
- Do something disagreeable that needs to be done by someone every day.
- Roll out of bed as soon as you awake after your planned hours of sleep. Make the decision the night before, and stick to it in the morning.
- Read deeply and thoughtfully, and stretch your mind to understand and retain what you read. Excessive reading of emotional fantasies weakens the will.
- The will is strengthened by exercise--self denial and self control. Practice denying yourself to pure indulgences especially when along.
- Link your will with Divine energy by asking God to empower your will.
- Practice healthful living with good nutrition, exercise, and rest.
- Make a habit of operating your life by plan, not impulse.

If you find it difficult to put any of the above exercises into practice, begin with the easiest until you have mastered it. Then take the next easiest, and so on. If it is still too difficult for you, try talking with God about it, and ask Him for His power to help you. When you have strengthen your will, you will truly be in charge of your life. Elden M Chalmers, Ph.D, Healing the Broken Brain, p. 25, 26.

Promoting Psychological Growth
Postulate 1. Prescription medicines may interfere with psychological growth.

Unfortunately, as is so often the case, even though the patient's initial response to the various medications seemed favorable, her physiological system soon adapted to each medication and shortly thereafter the tranquilizers acted upon her system like stimulants, and the anti-depressants like depressants. I remembered my psycho-pharmacology professor showing us slides from patient's charts that graphically described this reversing action of every stimulant, and every tranquilizer after prolonged use.

While such drug may be useful to remove an incapacitating symptom, most of them have harmful side effects. Some of these side effects threaten the user's life, weaken or destroy body and grain tissue, and upset the delicate chemical and electrical balance of our internal physical and mental process.

Principle: Any psychological value or technique that would contribute to high quality psychological health must contribute to quality growth.

Faith-Endurance-Patience
Faith: "Daughter be of good comfort; thy faith hath made thee whole, Matthew 9:22. There are many examples in scripture were Jesus told someone that their faith had healed them. What did Jesus mean by a person's faith healing them? What Jesus is saying is that the individual believed in Jesus Christ as the Messiah-the son of God; and if they died or lived, got sicker or healthier, they were content with the outcome because they trusted God. The individual believed that whatever item Jesus chooses to use to heal someone, i.e. mud and spittle, or just speak the words "rise, take up thy bed and walk" that it was blessed of God to heal them. When it comes to health restoration God's way, you have to believe in God and have faith in His way of healing, which is superior to man's system of sick care and be content with the outcome. Remember, "There are many ways of practicing the healing arts, but there is only one way that heaven approves" White, 5T, p. 443, (1885). What has God ordained as His remedies? "God's remedies are the simple agencies of nature that will not tax or debilitate the system through their powerful properties. Pure air and water, cleanliness, a proper diet, purity of life,

and a firm trust in God, are remedies for the want of which thousands are dying... 5T, Ellen White, p. 443, (1885).

Endurance: "...but he that shall endure unto the end, the same shall be saved", Matthew 13:13. As discussed earlier in the section Physically Reborn, true healing takes time. Most people do not want to put up with the pain or discomfort and immediately reach for the prescription medication, which gives them instant relief, but also lasting side-effects. It takes the right nutrients and the other laws of health to produce the next generation of healthy cells. "And so, after he had patiently endured, he obtained the promise, Hebrews 6:15.

Patience: "But let patience have her perfect work..." James 1:4. God said it and I believe it, therefore it is settled. If you will patiently follow God's Ten Laws of Health, not cheating yourself, then your faith in God and His healing methodology will reward your efforts. "...in which it was impossible for God cannot lie"..., Hebrews 6:18. True health is found by following the prescription for healing found in Isaiah 58:1-8.

Faith, hope, and love contribute to neuro-chemicals balance and health of mind.

Faith, hope, and love are examples of resources for growth. They also qualify as underlying principles for psychological health. Studies reported by Jeanne Achterberg and Frank Lawlis, [1/64] Joan Borysenko, [2/65] and others show how negative thinking is an example of one kind of experience that tends to destroy. Misdirected hate, envy, greed, generalized pugnacity are other examples. [3/66, 4/67]

When people exercise faith, their immune system rallies, wiping out destructive foreign invaders. At the same time, the faith flowing neuro-chemical pathways shut down the pathways that would trigger debilitating doubt. Genuine faith is not unreasonable. Repeatedly Jesus healed people so that they might believe that He also has power to forgive them.[5/68] Faith is our conviction about realities that we cannot see[6/69], and this conviction must be founded upon knowledge, a knowledge based upon the Word of God[7/70]. As a means of developing a transforming and enduring faith, there is no substitute for the regular and earnest study of the King James Bible. Chalmers Ph.D. TBB, p. 65.

The Nature and Power of Love

There is no fear in love; but perfect love casts our fear, because fear involves torment. But he who fears has not been made perfect in love."[8/71]

"Love suffereth long, *and* is kind; love envieth not; love vaunteth not itself, is not puffed up, Doth not behave itself unseemly, seeketh not her own, is not easily provoked, thinketh no evil; Rejoiceth not in iniquity, but rejoiceth in the truth; Beareth all things, believeth all things, hopeth all things, endureth all things. Love never faileth: [9/72]

Brain chemicals are secreted in just the right amounts and in the right locations. Here is one example: the brain chemical *oxytocin* secreted in abundance in the frontal lobe as evidenced by the abundance of *oxytocin* receptors found there is associated with *true love and fidelity*. When we activate and strengthen those true love pathways in the frontal lobe, a whole array of destructive emotions are held in check, -destructive hate, envy, fear, greed, sexual promiscuity, marital, infidelity, spousal and child abuse, --to cite a few! These are findings of neurological and psychological studies. I see such scientific data as the handwriting of God in human nature, often clarifying previously recorded revelations in the Bible.

Principle: Faith, hope, and love are essential to quality psychological healing. We need to promote positive psychological growth. Our psychological health depends on it.

Postulate 2. The Brain is Prepared for Repair and Growth.

The brain has the ability to adapt and change. We are not necessarily
victims of our genetics. We are not necessary the victims of a bad start in life. Our destiny is not necessarily determined by the hands of those who shaped us during the first few years of our life. We need not be the permanent victims of our own bad choices and practices. Even when large areas of the brain are missing because of birth defect, injury, or disease, the brain recognizes this loss and is prepared to develop the lost capacities in the brain area that remain. For example, an individual teaching themselves to talk or walk, etc… after a stroke.

We need to take responsibility for those aspects of our lives that we can do something about. As the apostle Paul put it, "Forgetting those things that are behind, and reaching forward to those things which are ahead"[10/73] –we can take responsibility for our choice of lifestyle—our nutrition, our exercise program, our rest times, our use of fresh air and pure water, our attitudes, our values, our habits, our priorities, our goals. We know that all of these affect the healthy functioning of our brain.

Again, we must not punish ourselves for the occasional neglect or sinful indulgence—these may mete out their own punishment,[11/74] but the occasional neglect or sinful indulgence does not establish habits in our brain networks, nor do they determine our character.[12/75] Let's not worry about past wrong-doing! We cannot unscramble eggs!

Postulate 3. Internal Harmony Means Psychological Health.

Purity of purpose and integrity are essential foundation principles

underlying the harmonious interaction of one's internal resources. They bring peace and calm to the mind and emotions. The energy of the brain is most productive and most efficient when there is harmony inside of us. Anxious people can find peace by:
1) Examining how they are using their internal resources,
2) making the decision to be true to the values of purity and integrity,
3) renouncing all contaminating influences,
4) using their talents and internal resources harmoniously i.e. in ways that are not in conflict, and
5) keeping their mind stayed on the Lord.

The approaches a therapist uses will vary from client to client and from therapist to therapist. A psychologically healthy therapist can adapt more readily to a wider variety of patient types, using approaches that best fit the patient. Christian therapist would do well to practice the biblical counsel in this regard.

"And of some have compassion, making a difference: And others save with fear, pulling them out of the fire; hating even the garment spotted by the flesh. Jude 1:22, 23.

Whatever course is followed, the goal of healing therapy is to mobilize our internal resources for *harmonious* action.

Postulate 4. The Growing Edge is the Healing Edge.

Psychological growth begins at the growing edge of our psychological self. We are defining the "growing edge" as the *healthy* perception, attitude, emotion, or personality characteristic that exists beneath any unhealthy expressions. Unless our unhealthy characteristics are removed and our healthy characteristics are nurtured, we will continue to make poor judgments in life.

Corollary #1: In order for growth to take place, the growing edge must be identified.

Corollary #2: Our unhealthy defenses must be removed, much as disease tissue must be removed in the surgical field, before new healthy tissue can grow. *Denial, blame, learned helplessness, and causeless ill-directed anger* are examples of unhealthy defenses that must be removed before the growing edge can be found.

To remove 'diseased psychological tissue', some therapists are comfortable with only one method-*confrontation*. These are instances in which "diseased tissue" is best dealt with in this manner. "Cry aloud, spare not; show my people their transgressions."[13/102] At other times, the disease tissue is best handled by bringing "*comfort*" to the client. "Comfort, yes, comfort My people! Speak comfort." [14/103] Still at other times, therapist must simply withhold what they would like to share with the client simply because the client cannot handle it at that time. "I still have many things to say to you, but you cannot bear them now." [15/104] The most helpful therapist will select from a variety of approaches the approach that best fits the client and the task at hand. The task in this instance is the removal of diseases tissue to discover the growing edge.

Preventing Psychological Breakdown

Postulate 5: A Healthy Brain Maintains Emotional Stability.

It was the American physician Walter B. Cannon who coined the term 'homeostasis in his book Wisdom of the Body, 1932. Cannon set forth the basic idea of feedback as a fundamental physiological principle. He explained that homeostasis is maintained by feedback signals from what is needed to how that need can be attained. This is an important principle for the guiding of skilled behavior, for making appropriate decisions and for guiding appropriate actions to satisfy our motivational and emotional needs.

Principle: In order for us to maintain emotional stability, our emotional centers must send feedback signals from the needy centers to the brain centers that can meet those needs.

Just as the principle of homeostasis operates in the physical self for the maintenance of a relatively stable environment, e.g. body temperature, so this principle operates in the psychological self. Homeostasis in the *psychological* self is its predisposition to maintain stability among contending motivations and other psychodynamic forces. The healthy psychological self adjusts homeostatically to prevent extreme departures from a comfortable *internal psychological* environment. Glands and organs throughout the brain and body are constantly supplying appropriate hormones and chemicals to maintain physiological and psychological homeostasis or stability. Flows of neural current trigger the release of appropriate chemicals in just the right amounts. Neuroscience has demonstrated that feedback and forward circuitry make homeostasis possible. We have learned that emotional homeostasis is the result of feedback and feed-forward neurological firing patterns.

Postulate 6: Temperance Protects from Psychological Breakdown.

Sometimes translated "self-control," "temperance"[16/105] typically means the moderate use and practice of anything helpful, and total abstinence from anything harmful. Intemperate stimulation or deprivation, intemperate rewards or punishment, obsessive rehearsals, compulsive rituals, fanatical pursuits of all kinds, "all work and no play" or vice-versa, and intemperance of all kinds prevent the development of true psychological health. They stress the brain and body efforts to

maintain harmony in the chemical secretions that flow in and out of nerve, gland, and organ. In addition, extremes push the brain to set up new reference standards for "typical" or "regular"
operations. In other words, in an attempt to handle the extreme situation, the new reference standards will become the "norm" for the brain. In the future, the person will tend to depend upon extremes to avoid boredom in life.

Postulate 7: Psychological Addictions cause the Breaks of your Brain to fail.

Generally speaking, the *unperverted* appetite can depend on "tissue hunger" dictating their tastes for the foods containing the appropriate nutrients. One study with 2-3 year old infants showed that infants could select a balanced diet by themselves if there was no refined sugar in any of their food![17/108] In another study, two scientist demonstrated that food intake tends to vary with changes in bodily needs for a particular substance. Rats deprived of their adrenal glands drank much heavier salt solutions than rats that had intact functioning adrenal glands. [18/109]

I repeated this study, adding a sugar solution to the options available to the rats. I discovered even though the adrenalectomized rats initially showed a distinct preference for the salt solution needed for survival, after just a few samplings of the sugar solution, they neglected the essential salt solution and showed their preference for the sugar solution. Even though, without their adrenal glands, they needed the salt solution to survive! Sugar can apparently pervert the appetite even when your life is at stake! [19/110]

Unfortunately, sometimes our imperfect bodies send us appetite signals of genuine tissue hunger that appear to be a perverted hunger, when in fact a defective gland or organ may be signaling the need for a nutrient in unusual amount. The following case sadly illustrates this reason for "tissue hunger". A three-year old boy hated anything sweet but craved anything salty. He not only licked the salt off the crackers and other foods, but on one occasion he climbed onto the kitchen counter to procure the salt shaker put "out of his reach" by his concerned parents, and was observed to consume nearly the entire contents of the salt shaker! Ultimately his parents were putting an excessive amount of salt on his food simply to get him to eat his food. The parents finally brought him to the hospital for other problems. On the well-regulated diet of the hospital, the three-year-old died within a week. An autopsy showed that his adrenal glands were defective. This defect had caused his body to lose salt faster than it was possible to replace on a normal diet.[20/111] When the nerves are robbed of their needed nutrients, the balancing of the inhibitory and excitatory pathways of the nervous system is disrupted. Psychological health cannot then be achieved. Anyone dealing with nerve disorders knows how long it takes for nerves to heal. There are no quick fixes for shattered nerves! Let's get beyond merely treating symptoms. Let's try to help nerves to experience true healing. Every little effort helps.

Postulate 8: Distributing the Workload of your Brain Protects it from Breakdown.

We have two brains: a left and a right. Both are chemically and structurally different. Modern brain scientists tell us that our left brain is our expressive brain—using letters, words, and numbers. It analyzes, organizes, and expresses itself. Our right brain is our receptive brain—receiving patterns, pictures, complex wholes, dreams, visions, aspirations, and intuitions. It sees the whole picture and does not try to analyze it.

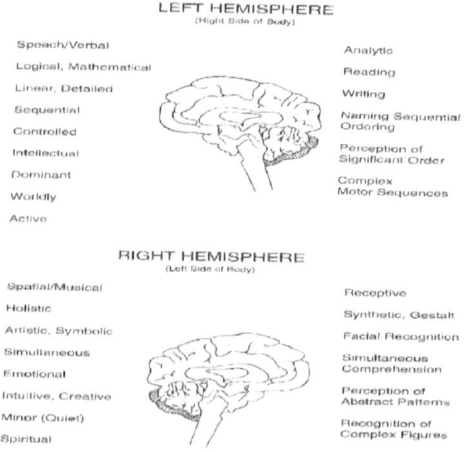

Our genetic code may have programmed the richness of development in certain areas of our brain, providing us with certain natural talents. It is natural to pursue that which comes easiest. By working to develop a talent that we do not naturally posses, we stimulate the growth and development of new areas of the brain. In this way, we can "acquire" a talent we did not have. God created us all to multiply the talents He has given us.[21/112] If we all worked to develop a facility in the use of both brains, we would be less likely to overwork any one area of the brain to the neglect of many other areas. Fatigue is a signal for changing our particular activity. Mental fatigue usually disappears with a little physical exercise activating the brain's motor strip and its pathways. Or it may disappear with a shift in the kind of mental activity engaged in. For example, number crunching interspersed with music or art. Many people pursue a very narrow range of activities. Many carry their work with them wherever they go. This work places heavy demands on the limited area of their brain. The result will be an imbalance in the secretion of the hormones and chemicals needed for healthy brain function.

The balanced use of our brain is vital for mental and emotional health. We need to practice exercises requiring the use of little used areas of the brain. By establishing a hierarchy of exercises, and beginning with the easiest until each becomes natural, we are more easily motivated to develop balance in the use of the mental powers.

Nurturing the Healing Process
Postulate 9: The Reactance Principle awakens the brain to Truth.

Most people in a relationship, marital or otherwise that have almost daily interaction with another person can begin to forget their good qualities and it is not until they are confronted with their extreme position that the *reactance principle* comes into play. They only see the other individual as bad, and treat them that way. At the same time they would be expressing the worse side of herself in anger, anxiety, frustration, and even depression over what would seem to them as a "*hopeless*" situation.

It is natural for us to see our situation as extreme. This defends our extreme emotions, our rash words and reckless actions. In fact spilt brain studies show that we have a remarkable way of justifying or rationalizing our careless words or actions. Psychologist Michael Gazzaniga believes the brain is organized into somewhat independent units that work on the same problem. According to his theory, the brain tends to by-pass those modules that contain the truth that contradicts our actions. When these "truth" modules are by-passed we are not aware of the whole truth. Furthermore, Leon Festinger's *cognitive dissonance* theory had previously led to studies testing Festinger's theory. These *cognitive dissonance* studies found that indeed doesn't like *dissonance*. The brain does not like it when our actions don't match our beliefs. And listen to this. These studies have found that if our actions continue to contradict our beliefs, we will change our beliefs to match our actions, -- not our actions to match our beliefs! In the mean time, according to Gazzaniga, the brain simply by-passes the modules that would show up our dysfunctional words and actions! If this is true, it would explain why we do not even recognize our own dysfunctionality!

If we find ourselves acting in such a dysfunctional manner, it is often helpful to write a letter to the offending person, read it over, talk to the Lord about it, and throw it away. Or re-write it to express our perceptions more accurately. It is easier for us to recognize how extreme our position is when we write it down, and re-read it. Remember, when we act as though life for us is all bad, our brain is probably by-passing the truth modules to make our beliefs match our actions.

Postulate 10: Awakening the Trace of a Divine Creation Brings Healing.[22/113]

A war is raging within—the war between the desire for goodness and the inclination to badness, between the perception of right and the perceived attractiveness of wrong. This creates an internal restlessness, confusion, and neurotic conflicts. We need to explore the likely outcomes of following the options available on both sides in "the war that rages within", and encourage the nurturing of the better self. We may need to take a walk, breathe deeply, and crystallize what our best self would do if we gave it some support.

We each possess intellectual power, spiritual power, the ability to know what is right, the desire for goodness, and our unique combinations of individualistic and positive qualities. We need to acknowledge the Source of these qualities and thank a loving Creator God for creating these within us. The nurturing of our impatience for whatever 'feels' good is an encouragement to emotional immaturity—the level that every child would operate on, namely the immediate gratification of the senses. These are precursors to the development of anti-social personalities.[23/114] Followed in early childhood; this practice of doing what initially feels good has been highly correlated with the development of children without a conscience.[24/115]

It is better to encourage ourselves to follow through on our deepest desires for goodness, do the right thing, and nurturing our spiritual power. We will soon experience "good feelings" that are not transient, but enduring. Thank God for these good feelings and for the privilege of fellowship with Him. I have found God quick to respond and energize those positive gifts He has blessed us with. These positive resources, i.e. desires for goodness, perception of right and spiritual power, will continue to increase and then multiply. They will gain new positive resources. They will be making long strides in the journey towards genuine mental and emotional health. Go back and review Dr. Trust in God from earlier in the book. For a read of all forty of Dr. Chalmers Postulates and Principles get a copy of his book "Healing the Broken Brain, Remnant publications.

Chapter IX: The Body Temple

God Dwells in you, His Living Temple: The Lord has graciously revealed to His children how important an understanding of the Sanctuary and its services are to our salvation and health is. It is so important that God gives us a clue of how to know Him in Psalms 77:13.

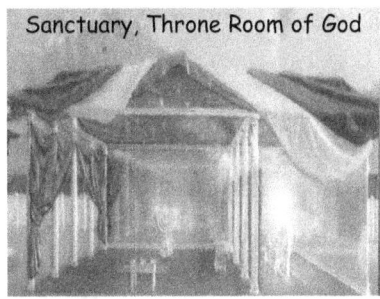

Sanctuary, Throne Room of God

"Thy way, O God, *is* in the sanctuary: who *is so* great a God as *our* God? Hebrews 8:2 tells us that our elder brother Jesus Christ is a Minister of the sanctuary and of the true tabernacle, in heaven that the Lord pitched and not man. We are also told in verse 5, that Moses was admonished to make the tabernacle on earth "according to the pattern shewed to thee in the mount". You can read about the earthly sanctuary and its services in the book of Leviticus, especially chapter 26. In I Corinthians 6:19, God makes a statement of almost disbelief, that you His professed child do not know that He dwells in you.

"What? Know ye not that your body is the temple of the holy ghost which is in you. Which ye have of God, and ye are not your own? For ye are bought with a price: therefore glorify God in your body, and in your spirit, which are God's". 1 COR. 6:19.

Not just God but every piece of furniture in the heavenly sanctuary dwells in you as well. He is God; therefore He has to have a throne room in you. Remember, He admonished Moses to make it according to the pattern.

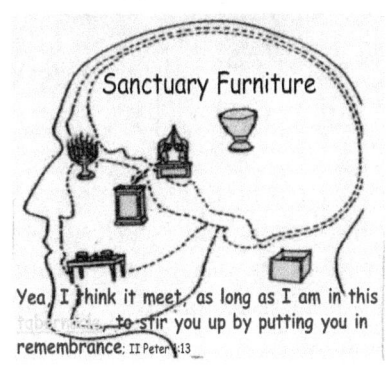

Sanctuary Furniture

Yea, I think it meet, as long as I am in this tabernacle, to stir you up by putting you in remembrance; II Peter 1:13

Greek Dictionary of the New Testament #4636: skenos: <u>a hut or temporary residence , i.e. the human body</u> (as the abode of the spirit);-<u>tabernacle</u>.

No wonder David exclaimed "I will praise thee; for I am fearfully *and* wonderfully made: marvellous *are* thy works; and *that* my soul knoweth right well," Psalms 139:14.

As we study human anatomy and the earthly sanctuary, we see God, His way and His original plan to dwell in humanity.

The apostle Peter said "Yea, I think it meet, as long as I am in this <u>tabernacle</u>, to stir you up by putting you in remembrance; II Peter 1:13.

Let us study to see how God has placed the furniture of His sanctuary in the human habitation. The sanctuary is a miniature representation of God's throne room, read Revelation chapters 4 and 5 in your study time.

The structure of the sanctuary consisted of 48 boards in the building, read: Exodus 26:18, 20, 22, 23

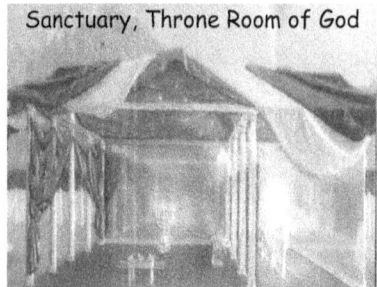
Sanctuary, Throne Room of God

1. 20 boards on the south side southward: Exodus 26:18
2. 20 boards on the north side: Exodus 26:20.
3. 6 boards westward: Exodus 26:22.
4. 2 boards for the corners of the Tabernacle in the two sides. Exodus 26:23-25. The total equals 48.

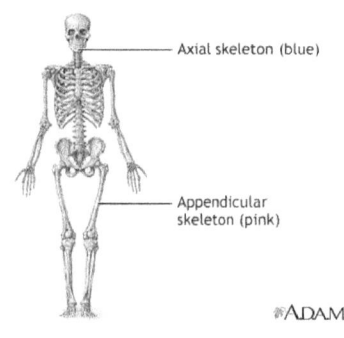

The supporting structure of the human anatomy consists of 24 Vertebrae's, & 24 Ribs coupled together in the central part of the axial skeleton. God used 48 items in the frame of both the sanctuary and human tabernacle to support the structure.

The sanctuary had 3 parts: the court yard, the holy place, and most holy place, representing the different parts of the head.

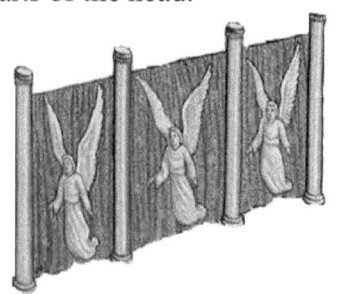

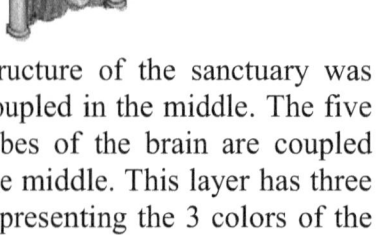

The Sanctuary Veil: And thou shalt make a veil of blue, and purple, and scarlet (red), and fine twined linen of cunning work: with cherubim shall it be made.... Exodus 26:31.

The structure of the sanctuary was coupled in the middle. The five lobes of the brain are coupled in the middle. This layer has three parts representing the 3 colors of the veil. Exodus 26:33.

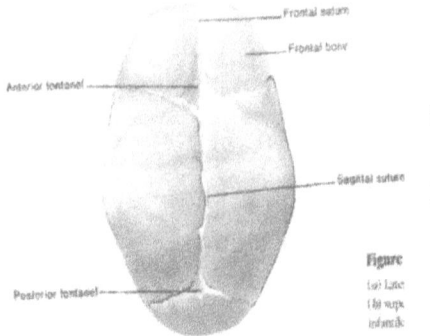

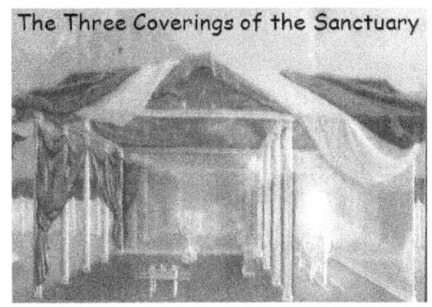
The Three Coverings of the Sanctuary

The Sanctuary had Three coverings: "And thou shalt make curtains of goats hair... Exodus 26:7 (white), and thou shalt make a covering for the tent of rams' skins dyed red ... Exodus 26:14, And a covering above of badgers' skin (black)... Exodus 26:14.

The body temple has the same three coverings as the sanctuary; 1). First layer is white bone, protecting the brain with the frontal lobe doubled at birth. 2). Next is a solid piece of scalp with no couplings, which contains many blood vessels. 3). the hair is the outside covering. God was very particular about the number so that it would truly represent the covering on the head.

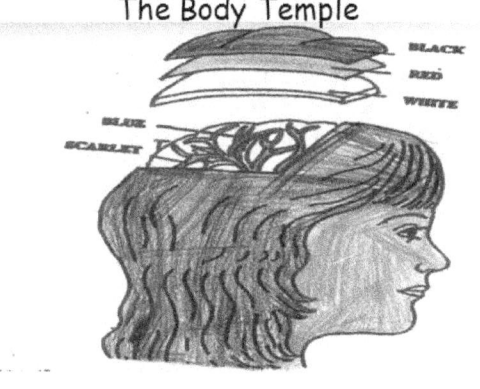
The Body Temple

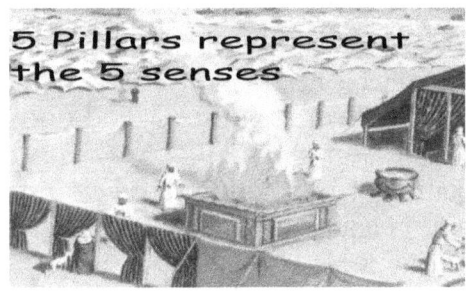
5 Pillars represent the 5 senses

There were 5 pillars holding the entrance curtain to the sanctuary. They represent the 5 senses of hearing, sight, taste, touch and smell; by which information is reported to the brain to be processed and become part of the character.

"Those who would not fall a prey to Satan's devices, must guard well the avenues of the soul; they must avoid reading, seeing, or hearing that which will suggest impure thoughts. The mind must not be left to dwell at random upon every subject that the enemy of souls may suggest. The heart must be faithfully sentineled, or evils without will awaken evils within, and the soul will wander in darkness. The body is

The 5 Avenues to the Soul

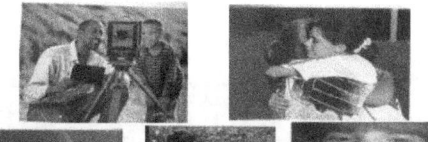
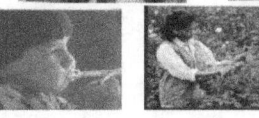
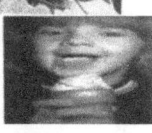

the only medium through which the mind and the soul are developed for the up building of character. Hence it is that the adversary of souls directs his temptations to the enfeebling and degrading of the physical powers. His success here means the surrender to evil of the whole being. The tendencies of our physical nature, unless under the dominion of a higher power, will surely work ruin and death." E.G. White, Counsel on Diets and Foods, p.73.

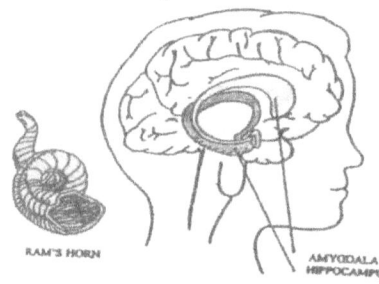

Shofar; Trumpet or Ram's Horn

The trumpet that was used to call the people to the sanctuary was called the Shafer, a ram's horn. It was used to bring to remembrance the instructions – a call to worship, to war, to march, a warning, etc. This part of the brain is involved in memory and emotions. You had to remember the different signals. Imagine the emotion when Jesus comes and we hear the trump of God 1 Thess. 4:13-17.

It is ordained by God, according to the Plan of Salvation, divinity and humanity must work together. *"As soon as we consent to give up sin, to acknowledge our guilt, the barrier is removed between the soul and the savior."* Selected Messages, bk 1, p. 325.

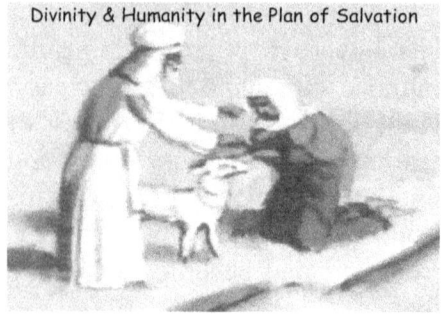

Divinity & Humanity in the Plan of Salvation

If we confess our sins, he is faithful and just to forgive us [our] sins, and to cleanse us from all unrighteousness, I John 1:9. "Whosoever is born of God doth not commit sin; for his seed remaineth in him: and he cannot sin, because he is born of God" 1 John 3:9.

The alter of sacrifice was the first thing seen when entering the courtyard. It represents the sacrifice of the Lamb of God upon the cross. "Behold the lamb of God which taketh away the sins of the world" (John 1:29).

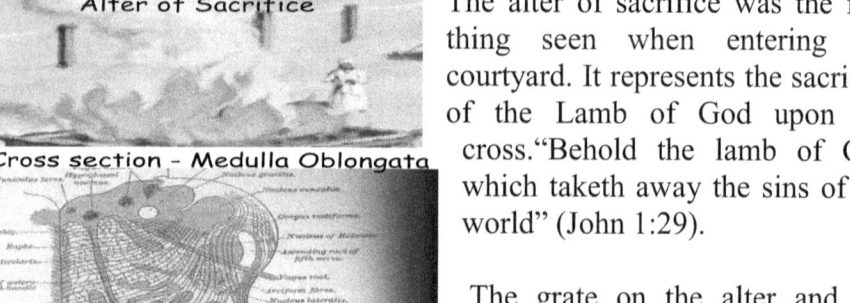

Alter of Sacrifice

Cross section - Medulla Oblongata

The grate on the alter and the table of showbread were the same height, as are the mouth and the medulla. When you slice the medulla, it looks like a grate. This part of the brain is involved in involuntary functions, such as respiration, heart rate, etc., that occur without conscious thought. Every since the fall of mankind, sin is practiced naturally, without conscious thought. The sacrifice of Christ was to change that process and make us a new creature, if we choose.

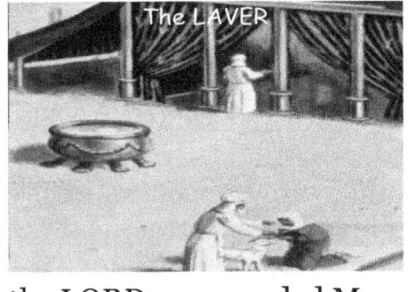

And he set the laver between the tent of the congregation and the altar, and put water there, to wash *withal*. And Moses and Aaron and his sons washed their hands when they went into the tent of the congregation, and when they came near unto the altar, they washed; as the LORD commanded Moses, Ex. 40: 30-32.

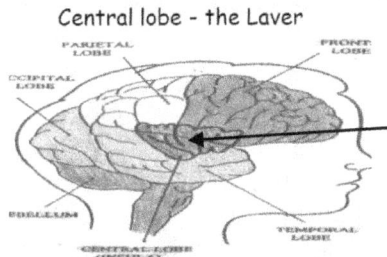

Buried under all the other lobes of the brain is the insula, which is especially protected. It lies deep within the folds of the lateral sulcus. Science has not fully discovered all the functions of this part of the brain, but it is shaped like a bowl laver).

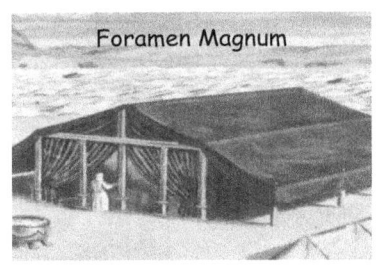

The priests and high priest went in and out of the curtain (foramen magnum) of the sanctuary receiving instructions from the Lord. The foramen magnum was the entry from the court yard into the holy place of the sanctuary.

In the picture on the left, you can see the opening in the Occipital Bone through which the spinal cord passes from the brain. The first structure upon entering the foramen magnum is the brainstem. This part of the brain is involved with involuntary functions such as respiration, heart rate, etc... that occur without conscious thought.

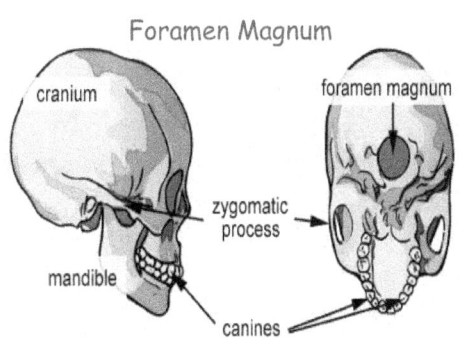

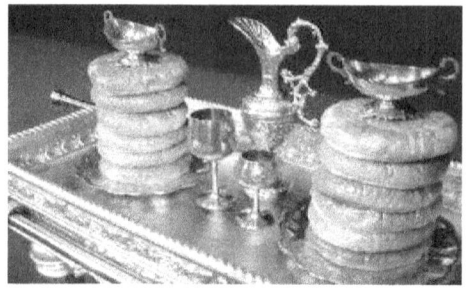

Eating the word of God

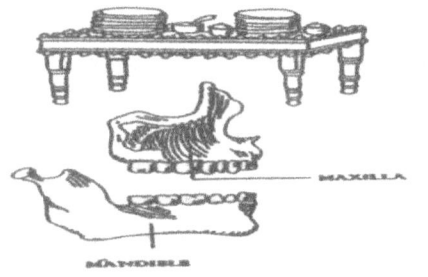

and thou shalt set upon the table shewbread before me always, Exodus 25:30.

And Jesus said unto them, "I am the bread of life..." John 6:35.

The table of showbread had a shelf with a crown, and a border of a hand's breadth with another crown. God was very specific in this instruction. The Bread is ingested through the mouth, where we have 2 sets of crowns, one on a wide bone, the other one on a narrow bone.

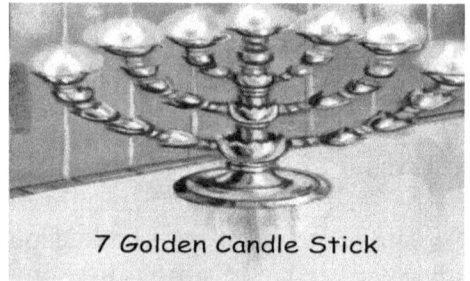

7 Golden Candle Stick

The candlestick was to give light in the sanctuary. It was never to go out, Lev. 24:4.
Read Zechariah 4 and note the similarity of the trees and pipes.

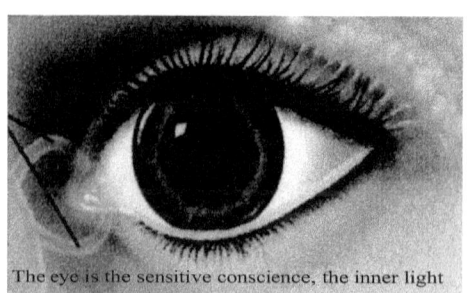

The eye is the sensitive conscience, the inner light

The eye is the sensitive conscience, the inner light, of the mind. Upon its correct view of things, the spiritual healthfulness of the whole soul and being depends. The "eye-salve,' the Word of God, makes the conscience smart under its application, for it convicts of sin. But the smarting is necessary that the healing may follow, and the eye be single to the glory of God. . . . Says Christ, by renouncing your own self-sufficiency, giving up all things, however dear to you, you may buy the gold, the raiment, and the eye-salve that you may see." White, Our High Calling, p. 350.

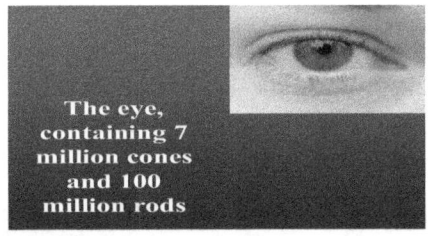

The eye contains seven million cones and one hundred million rods.

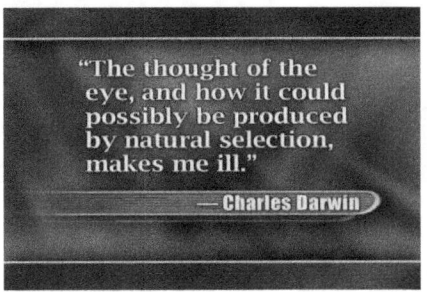

"The thought of the eye, and how it could possibly be produced by natural selection, makes me ill."
--Charles Darwin

Remember, we are discussing God's throne room in the human habitation. Showing each article of furniture in the earthly sanctuary as it corresponds with the same article of furniture in the human tabernacle, the abode of God the Holy Spirit. Both tabernacles are an exact pattern of the heavenly sanctuary.

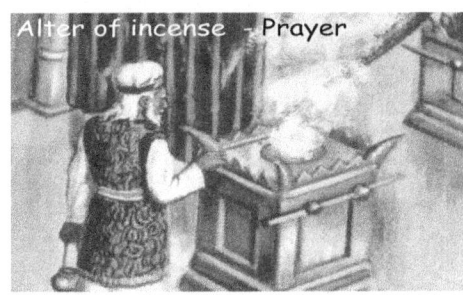

The Alter of Incense was the place of prayer. The incense had four spices plus salt, making five ingredients in all. Five is the number of grace and redemption and the smoke from the incense represented the merits of Jesus, which went up with the prayers of the saints. In order to make the incense, it had to be "beaten". In order to make the Shewbread it was kneaded, the candle stick and the incense were beaten, Ex. 25:31 and Lev. 16:12. This beating represented the beating Christ would subject Himself too.

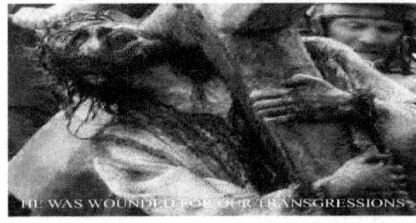

"But he was wounded for our transgressions; he was bruised for our iniquities: the chastisement of our peace was upon him; and with his stripes we are healed." Isaiah 53:5.

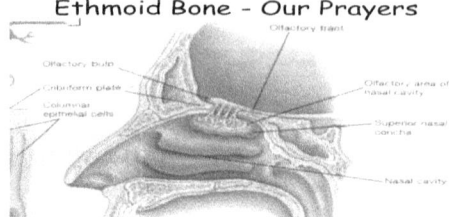
Ethmoid Bone - Our Prayers

The nerves of the sense of smell travel through the Ethmoid Bone to the Olfactory Bulbs. This is the only one of the five senses that is not routed through the Thalamus; it represents our prayers.

Thus your prayers are accepted, becoming unto God a sweet-smelling savor in the beloved. (Thus you enter into his rights, and become an heir with God and joint heir with Jesus Christ. You will enter into His victories, and the reward of eternal life will be given you. "But as many as received him, to them gave He power to become the sons of God, *even* to them that believe on his name: Which were born, not of blood, nor of the will of the flesh, nor of the will of man, but of God." Jn. 1:12.

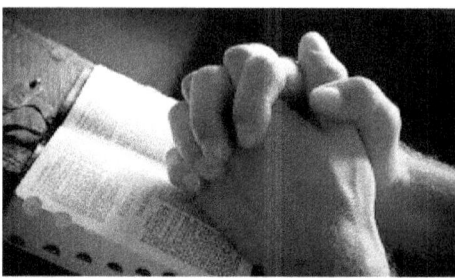

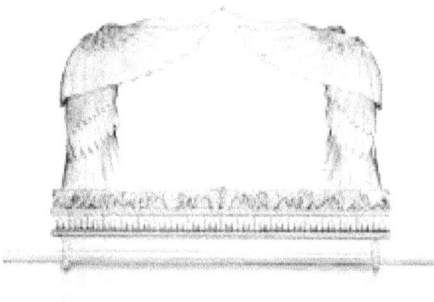
Ark of the Covenant

The Ark of the Covenant is located in the Most Holy place of the heavenly, earthly and human Sanctuary, it contains Manna (grain), Ex. 16:33, Almonds (nuts), Num. 17:8, pomegranates (fruit) Ex. 39:24, and God's 10 Commandment Law, the Mercy-Seat and His Holy Shekina.

The Sphenoid bone in the head represents the Ark of the Covenant. Because of its location and how it protects the content with in.

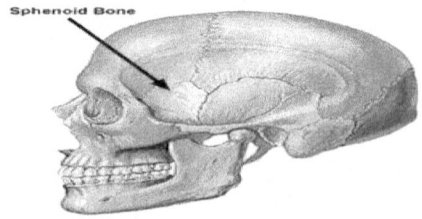

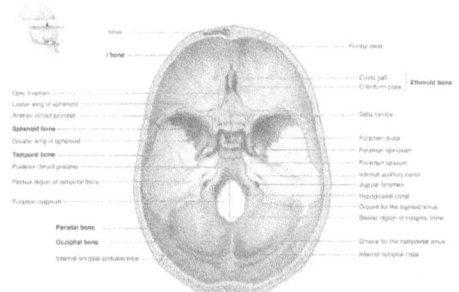

The Sphenoid bone touches all the bones of the head. Notice the wings, notice the box called the Sella Tursica. This is the space were the Pituitary gland sits. Over it is a membrane that represents the mercy seat.

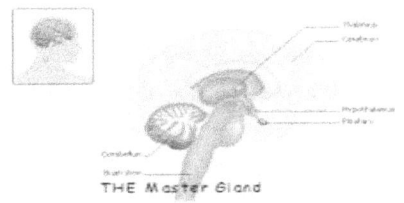
THE Master Gland

The Pituitary is the master gland; it has two working parts, —the anterior lobe, or adenohypophysis, and the posterior lobe, or neurohy-pophysis, which represents the two tables of the 10 Commandments.

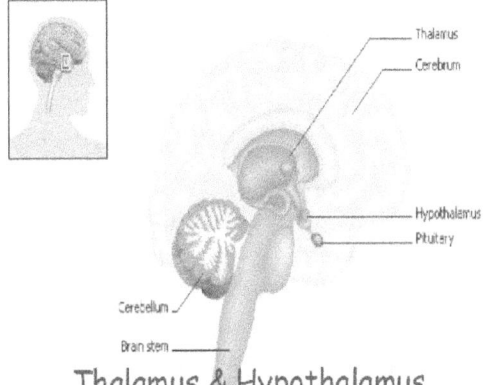
Thalamus & Hypothalamus

In the sanctuary the glory of God was manifested above the Ark of the Covenant in the most holy place. There are 8 nuclei in the hypothalamus; 8 is the special number of the Holy Spirit, the number of regeneration. There is 1 thalamus on each side. …"behold I see the heavens opened, and the Son of man standing on the right hand of God (acts 7:56).

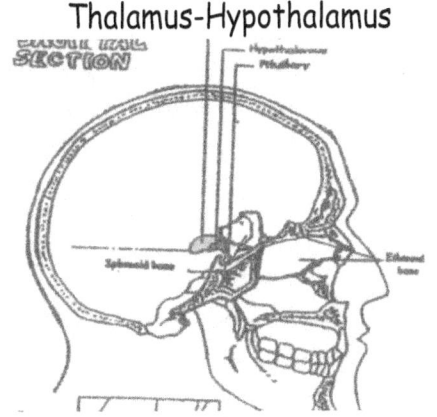
Thalamus-Hypothalamus

The three persons of the Godhead are represented here in the throne room of the brain. The thalamus (Jesus Christ) interprets and defines messages and passes instruction to the hypothalamus (Holy Spirit), John 16:13-15. Satan wanted to sit on this throne (Isa. 14:12-14).

"And I beheld, and I heard the voice of many angels round about the throne and beasts and the elders; and the number of them was ten thousand times ten thousand, and thousand of thousands;" Rev. 5:11. There were angels embroidered on the first covering of the sanctuary to impress the fact that angels are ever present to

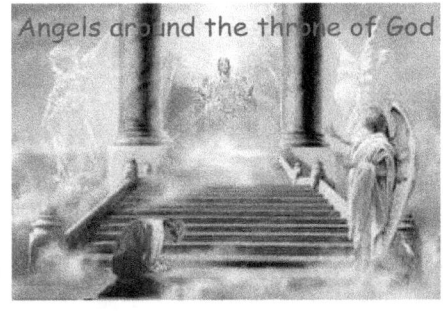
Angels around the throne of God

help us, Hebrews 1:14. You can read the description of the throne room of God in Revelation chapters 4 & 5.

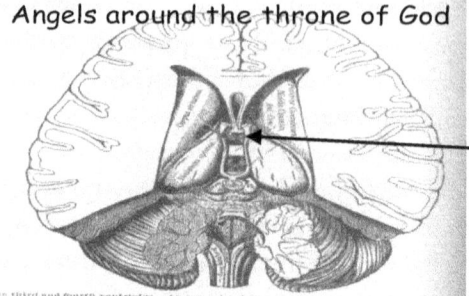

Angels around the throne of God

In this coronal view of the brain from Gray's Anatomy, the form of an angel wing is apparent. In the middle of the form of an angel is where the throne room of God is located in the brain.

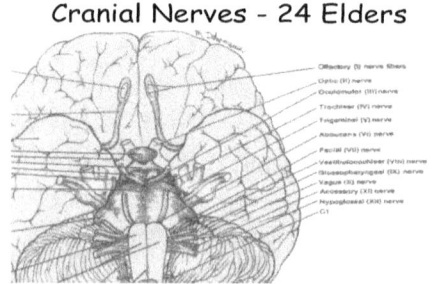

Cranial Nerves - 24 Elders

There are 12 cranial nerves on each side of your brain that help the brain to govern the body. They represent the 24 elders in Rev. 4 & 5. These people went with Jesus from the earth at the time of His ascension, Matt. 27:52, 53 and are helping in the Judgment in heaven. *"Those who came forth from the grave at Christ's resurrection were raised to everlasting life. They were the multitude of captives who ascended with Him as trophies of His victory over death and the grave. . . ."* Christ Triumphant, p. 286.2.

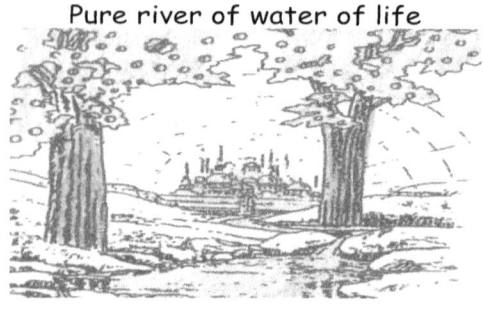

Pure river of water of life

"And he showed me a pure river of water of life, clear as crystal, proceeding out of the throne of God and of the Lamb. In the mist of the street of it, and on either side of the river, was there the tree of life, which bare 12 manner of fruits, and yielded her fruit every month: and the leaves of the tree were for the healing of the nations" Rev. 22; 1, 2. There was a tree on either side of the river but it came together as one tree at the top, just as the cerebellum contains 2 parts, but is joined in the middle. The spinal fluid runs between the two trees.

Cerebellum - Tree of Life

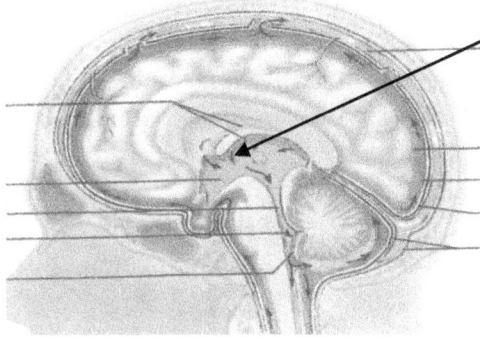

The spinal fluid originates in the ventricles in the throne room area of the brain, just as the river of life proceeds out of the throne of God, Rev. 22:1, 2. The spinal fluid must be pure or there will be major health problems, usually death.

Circulation of Cerebrospinal Fluid (CSF)

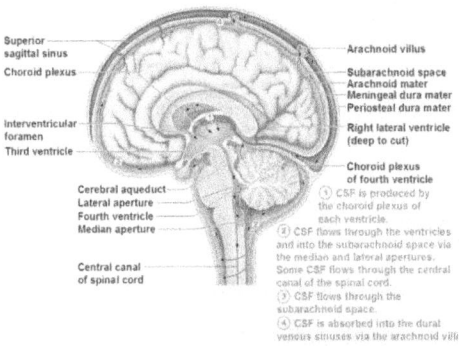

The spinal fluid runs down between the arbor vitae (medical term in Latin meaning tree of life) in the cerebellum, just as the river of life has the tree of life on either side.

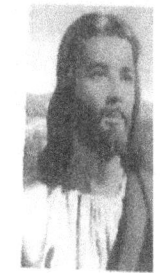

Their minds (frontal lobes) were given to God in this world; they served Him with their heart and intellect, and now He can put His name in their foreheads. He takes them as His children, saying, Enter ye into the joy of your Lord. The crown of immortality is placed on the brow of the over comers.

"And they shall see His face; and his name shall be in their foreheads."

Revelation 22:4

They take their crowns and cast them at the feet of Jesus, and touching their golden harps, they fill all heaven with rich music in songs of praise to the Lamb. Then "they shall see his face; and his name shall be in their foreheads." White, Our Father Cares, p. 142.2.

"Know ye not that ye are the temple of God, and that the spirit of God dwelleth in you? If any man defile the temple of God, him shall God destroy; for the temple of God is holy, which temple ye are." 1 COR. 3:16, 17.

Chapter X: God Heals Mental Diseases Naturally

What Is Depression?

Depression (major depressive disorder) is a common and serious medical illness that negatively affects how you feel the way you think and how you act. Fortunately, it is also treatable. Depression causes feelings of sadness and/or a loss of interest in activities once enjoyed. It can lead to a variety of emotional and physical problems and can decrease a person's ability to function at work and at home.

Depression symptoms can vary from mild to severe and can include:
- Feeling sad or having a depressed mood
- Loss of interest or pleasure in activities once enjoyed
- Changes in appetite — weight loss or gain unrelated to dieting
- Trouble sleeping or sleeping too much
- Loss of energy or increased fatigue
- Increase in purposeless physical activity (e.g., hand-wringing or pacing) or slowed movements and speech (actions observable by others)
- Feeling worthless or guilty
- Difficulty thinking, concentrating or making decisions
- Thoughts of death or suicide

Symptoms must last at least two weeks for a diagnosis of depression.

Also, medical conditions (e.g., thyroid problems, a brain tumor or vitamin deficiency and chronic dehydration) can mimic symptoms of depression so it is important to rule out general medical causes.

Depression affects an estimated one in 15 adults (6.7%) in any given year. And one in six people (16.6%) will experience depression at some time in their life. Depression can strike at any time, but on average, first appears during the late teens to mid-20s. Women are more likely than men to experience depression. Some studies show that one-third of women will experience a major depressive episode in their lifetime.

Depression Is Different From Sadness or Grief/Bereavement

The death of a loved one, loss of a job or the ending of a relationship are difficult experiences for a person to endure. It is normal for feelings of sadness or grief to develop in response to such situations. Those experiencing loss often might describe themselves as being "depressed." But being sad is not the same as having depression. The grieving process is natural and unique to each individual and shares some of the same features of depression. Both grief and depression may involve intense sadness and withdrawal from usual activities. They are also different in important ways:

- In grief, painful feelings come in waves, often intermixed with positive memories of the deceased. In major depression, mood and/or interest (pleasure) are decreased for most of two weeks.
- In grief, self-esteem is usually maintained. In major depression, feelings of worthlessness and self-loathing are common.
- For some people, the death of a loved one can bring on major
- Depression, losing a job or being a victim of a physical assault or a major disaster can lead to depression for some people. When grief and depression co-exist, the grief is more severe and lasts longer than grief without depression. Despite some overlap between grief and depression, they are different. Distinguishing between them can help people get the help, support or treatment they need.

Risk Factors for Depression

Depression can affect anyone—even a person who appears to live in relatively ideal circumstances.

Several factors can play a role in depression:
- **Biochemistry:** Differences in certain chemicals in the brain may contribute to symptoms of depression.
- **Genetics:** Depression can run in families. For example, if one identical twin has depression, the other has a 70 percent chance of having the illness sometime in life.
- **Personality:** People with low self-esteem, who are easily overwhelmed by stress, or who are generally pessimistic appear to be more likely to experience depression.
- **Environmental factors**: Continuous exposure to violence, neglect, abuse or poverty may make some people more vulnerable to depression. www.psychiatry.org/patients-families/depression/what-is-depression

What do we know about the safety of St. John's wort for depression?
- St. John's wort may limit the effectiveness of many prescription medicines.
- Combining St. John's wort and certain antidepressants can lead to a potentially life-threatening increase in your body's levels of serotonin, a chemical produced by nerve cells.

How God's Ten Doctors Heal Depression Naturally?

Depression is among the most treatable of mental disorders. Between 80 percent and 90 percent of people with depression eventually respond well to treatment. Almost all patients gain some relief from their symptoms. Before a diagnosis or treatment, a health professional should conduct a thorough diagnostic evaluation, including an interview and possibly a physical examination. In some cases, a blood test might be done to make sure the depression is not due to a medical condition like a thyroid problem. The evaluation is to identify specific symptoms, medical and family history, cultural factors and environ-mental factors to arrive at a diagnosis and plan a course of action.

Chapter XI: Herbs in the Laboratory:

Gingko Biloba

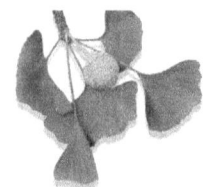

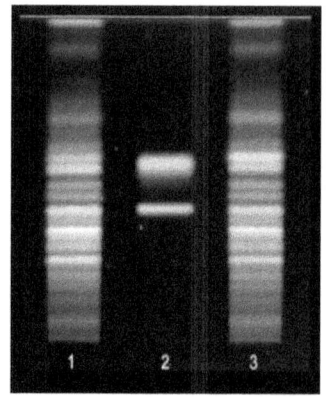

What is needed is a technology that really shows what herbs are really made up of. At a research center in Germany with its state of the art laboratory, scientist have discovered in recent years that it is possible to analysis plants in sort of details that Commission E researchers (Commission E Monographs) could have only dreamt of. The different lines represent a different chemical compound from the herb. Taking herbs apart like this means that we can see exactly what they are made of. So if you take a look at the finger print of the gingko leaf and you know how to read it, it is separated out into lots of different chemicals. Some of which are ginkgolides and they can help to prevent blood clots. Ginkgolides are a family of chemicals with known medicinal properties that are only found in ginkgo.

Hawthorne Leaf:

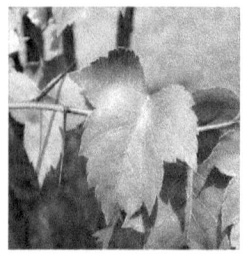

Hawthorne is supposed to be good for the cardiovascular system.
It contains polyphenols and can make your heart beat stronger. So
Is no question that herbs contain some useful chemicals, but it is not clear that they are in a form that the human body can absorb? In short, have the potential to work but that does not mean that they do. To answer that question they need to be tested on people.

Herbal Studies from Germany: St. John's wort

One of the most thoroughly investigated is an herb believed to relieve depression. Germany is one of the world's leading scientific research centers in the world on herbal remedies. Schwabe Pharmaceuticals was one of the first pharmaceutical companies in Germany to put St. John's wort under the microscope and conduct human trials. The testing and studies were based upon the fact that Schwabe knew that there was strong antidotal and historical use for St. John's wort for people who were sadness, depression or rejected. "So what we wanted to know, was could we boast up this experience based knowledge by modern clinical trials." Dr. Stephan Koehler, Schwabe Pharmaceuticals. St. John's wort contains a chemical called hypericum perforatum, which is believed to reduce depression. But is it in a form that can be used by the human body? The researchers recruited nearly 2000 volunteers suffering from mild to moderate depression. Some of the volunteers were then given a standardized extract of St. John's wort. The rest got a conventional antidepressant or dummy pill. Over the course of the trials researchers carefully monitored the mental state of each

Volunteer. Then they analyzed the data. Would St. John's wort be effective? The results were unequivocal. "We found that there is a considerable amount gets completely cured. And what is very amazing is that many of these people do not get another episode again, it prevents them from relapsing." -- Dr. Stephan Koehler, Schwabe Pharmaceuticals.

In a more recent trial 50% of those who took St. John's wort improved, against just 33% who took a standard antidepressant. Moreover, twice as many of those on conventional drugs reported side effects.

Now, an Herbal Extract to Treat Depression:
Washington February 11, 2005 2:07
"A British Medical Journal study has suggested that a specially manufactured extract from the herb St. John's wort is at least as effective in treating depression as a commonly prescribed anti-depressant" (and without the side effects). WEBINDIA123.com
www.The Power of Herbs–Full Herbal Medicine Documentary–BBC

Backed by extensive scientific research especially from Germany where some 3 million prescriptions for hypericum and almost 66 million doses of hypericum preparations are consumed annually, this ancient botanical, the favorite of herbalists of present and centuries past, is beginning to catch on in North America as a treatment for this all too common disorder as well as other forms of nervous anxiety, and sleep disorders. To date, there have been numerous case reports and drug monitoring studies with more than 5000 patients on the efficacy and safety of standardized St John's wort preparations. Twenty three controlled double-blind studies have been conducted on more than 1757 patients. Sixteen of these compared hypericum with placebo (sugar-pills) and 9 with standard reference treatments including Imipramine-2, Amitryptilin-2, Maprotiline-1, Desipramine-1, Diazepam-2 and Light therapy. In most of these studies, both depressive symptoms (depressed mood, anxiety, loss of interest, feelings of low worth, decreased activity) together with secondary symptoms (sleep disturbance, lack of concentration, bodily complaints such as fatigue) showed a general clinical improvement ranging from 50 to 80% when compared to that of low to medium dose treatment with "classic" synthetic antidepressants .

In another German study on 3,250 patients (76% women and 24% men), recorded by 663 private practitioners, the proportion of improvement in depressive and secondary physical symptoms (ranging from fatigue, cardiac, digestive and sleep disorders, to generalized pains) is similar to the previous studies with about 80% of all patients feeling better and only 15% unchanged or worse when asked an overall judgment. In these studies hypericum extracts were significantly superior to placebo and similarly effective as standard antidepressants (about 80%) with significantly fewer side effects than standard antidepressant drugs.
https://planetherbs.com/specific-herbs/treating-depression-with-st-johns-wort.html

A 2008 review of 29 international studies suggested that St. John's wort may be better than a placebo and as effective as different standard prescription antidepressants for major depression of mild to moderate severity. St. John's wort also appeared to have fewer side effects than standard antidepressants. The studies conducted in German-speaking countries—where St. John's wort has a long history of use by medical professionals—reported more positive results than those done in other countries, including the United States.
https://nccih.nih.gov/health/stjohnswort/sjw-and-depression.htm

If you read the research papers from not just German speaking countries but Traditional Chinese Medicine (TCM) and Ayurvedic Medicine, and the countries in the east, report favorable results treating depression alternatively than do their western counterparts. Remember, it was another western governmental agency, the FDA that has taken L-Tryptophan off the market and is only available via prescription, which is available through Original Healing Ltd. It is your body, your health and your life, both physically and spiritually now and possibly hereafter. As this book is written from a Christian perspective with Christians as the main target audience, remember it is the frontal lobe that you have to protect at all cost if you want to experience eternal life. Trust in God to heal you naturally and if He chooses not and allow you to sleep the sleep of death, then you have brought glory to His name by using His 10 health doctors that you might obtain a better resurrection.

Chapter XII: Rigorous Herbal Clinical Trials

Today after rigorous clinical trials we know certain herbs do work. There is overwhelming scientific evidence that what are called the super herbs works medicinally.

St. John's wort for mild to moderate depression,

Black Cohosh combats some of the affects of menopause,

Devil's Claw acts as an anti-inflammatory and can help with joint pain

Garlic can reduce cholesterol and decrease your blood pressure,

Saw Palmetto can relieve enlarged prostate,

Hawthorne leaf can help with some heart conditions, and

Horse Chestnuts improve poor blood circulation in the leg, helping some of the symptoms of varicose veins,

Ginkgo improves memory and other cognitive functions,

These herbs and some others are proven to work. They have been through clinical trials that are just as rigorous as those used for conventional drugs.

What is causing real excitement in the scientific and herbal community is not that herbs work but how they work. Scientist in South Africa has been looking into how herbs work. At the University of Johannes Berg, Dr. Carl Albrecht, Biochemist has isolated certain molecules from a particular herb. He has isolated a group of chemicals known as flavonoids. They contain chemicals structures that are proven, highly relevant pharmacological activity on cancer cells and HIV, the mystery is how do they get into the cell?

What's puzzling is that flavonoids are very large molecules, so large that they do not easily pass through a cell's membrane. So they should be impossible for the human body to absorb.

Dr. Albrecht wondered if he missed something. The interesting thought that has arisen in our research is that there is another family of molecules called satinens, or the detergents, a soap like molecules. When Dr. Albrecht put some of the plant material into a bleaker of water and shook it up, a soap layer was seen on top of the water. So the idea that arose, couldn't it be that these satinens are acting on the membrane of the cells to change the structure of the membrane to allow the flavonoids to go through. In short what makes herbs so special is that unlike conventional drugs, it is not a single chemical, it is a cocktail of chemicals that react together so that the sum is greater than the part. It is a process called synergy. You might think of it as an orchestra with each of the different instruments working together. Unfortunately, symphony's of chemicals like this is still too complicated for scientists to reproduce. Yet, there is tantalizing evidence that it is precisely this cocktail that give herbs that gives herbs their special healing powers.

On place that they are testing this ideal is London's Imperial College. Here they are examining whether a herbal cocktail can be exploited to treat one of the most puzzling chronic conditions of the 21 century, Alzheimer! The research is being lead by Dr. James Warner.

Alzheimer: Like all types of dementia, Alzheimer's is caused by brain cell death. It is a neurodegenerative disease, which means there is progressive brain cell death that happens over a course of time. The total brain size shrinks with Alzheimer's - the tissue has progressively fewer nerve cells and connections. Apr 29, 2016. Alzheimer's disease is caused by parts of the brain shrinking (atrophy), which affects the structure and function of particular brain areas. It's not known exactly what causes this process to begin. However, in the brains of people with Alzheimer's disease, scientists have found amyloid plaques (abnormal deposits of protein), neurofibrillary tangles (containing tau) and imbalances in a chemical called acetylcholine. It's also common to have a degree of vascular damage in the brain. These reduce the effectiveness of healthy neurons (nerve cells that carry messages to and from the brain), gradually destroying them. Over time, this damage spreads to several areas of the brain. The first areas affected are responsible for memories. The problem for doctors is that there is no clear understanding of what causes this multiple degeneration. There are a number of different theories, one of them is which there may be a chemical called free-radicals attacking the brain tissue. There is another possibility which is that the blood vessels in people with Alzheimer's disease begin to narrow, this causes an interruption of the blood supply to the brain and as a result, brain cells die.

So it seems that several different things are all contributing to Alzheimer's. And it is this very complexity that has made attempts to treat it using conventional drugs relativity unsuccessful. The difficulty is that creating medicines that can tackle several causes at one time is extremely difficult. Yet, according to Dr. Warner, there is an herbal cocktail that might be capable of doing just that. It's that remarkable plant Ginkgo. It is an extraordinary complex mixture of up to 200 chemicals. This means that unlike conventional drugs, it may be able to have several different affects simultaneously. The great advantage of ginkgo is that. this. Nearly all conventional medicines are single chemical entities. They usually only have one action, were as ginkgo has many actions. In other words, it is the herbal shotgun that can hit a range of targets versus the conventional single bullet that can only hit one. But is Dr. Warner right? To find out, he is running what he hopes will be the definitive clinical trial into whether ginkgo can help with Alzheimer's. Nearly 200 volunteers suffering from varying degrees of Alzheimer's have been recruited. Each has been assessed and then given ginkgo or a dummy pill; then revisited six months later and reassessed to see if there has been any change. Earlier trails have shown success and this trial could have much wider implications. May just be that like Alzheimer's many of the chronic diseases of the 21 century require a more complex chemical cocktail than modern medicine can currently make. In which case, herbs in all their complexity may just be the answer.

What is now clear is that when the FDA or a Pharmeuctical company runs lab test on a particular herb, the question becomes how was the lab test conducted? Was the specific chemical in question isolated, or was it tested with the necessary chemical(s) in order for it to be accepted into and active inside the human body?

Chapter XIII: Dr. Hoffer's M.D. Natural Schizophrenia Protocol

"For schizophrenia, the recovery rate with drug therapy is under 15%. With nutritional therapy, the recovery rate is 80%."

--Dr. Abram Hoffer **M.D.**

- Vitamin C   1g TID
- B complex   1g TID
- Niacin to tolerance 3-9mg TID
    - Take right after finishing a meal

Suggested
- B6 (pyridoxine)   250mg   QD
- Zinc citrate   50mg   QD

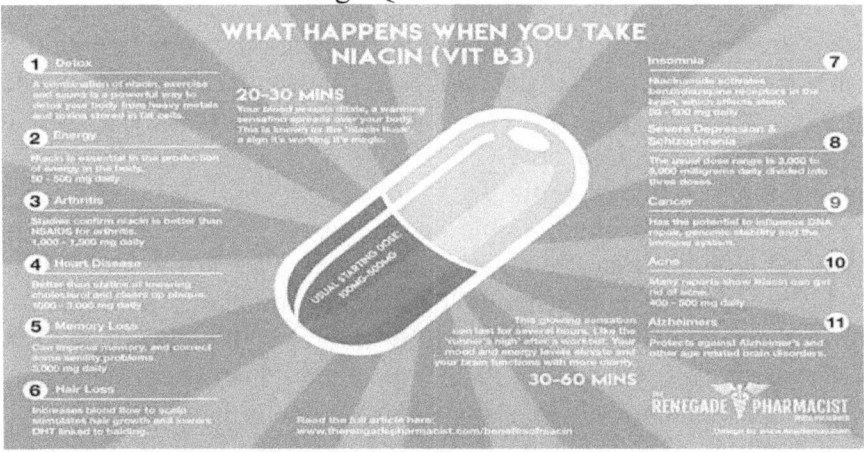

Dr. Abram Hoffer **M.D** Diet For schizophrenia

Dr. Hoffer advocated a vegetarian diet. I believe Dr. Hoffer was advocating a vegan diet because in his day and times there were only two definitions, meat eater or non-meat eater (vegetarian). Today, we have vegetarian, vegan, pescatarian, and many other names to define individual tastes.

Dairy Free
- What other species drinks another species milk?
- What species continues to drink milk after it has been weaned?

Refined Sugar Free
- No refined and/or processed Sugars
- limit sweeteners: Agave, honey & Maple Syrup

FOR IMMEDIATE RELEASE
Orthomolecular Medicine News Service, December 2, 2017

Niacin Treatment of Schizophrenia
Recent Research Confirms Abram Hoffer's Original Work,
by Robert G. Smith, PhD

(OMNS Dec 2, 2017) Schizophrenia is a devastating and complex disease that can include a variety of specific clinical conditions. Drugs to treat schizophrenia have not advanced much beyond the 1960s; in many cases they are not very effective, and they have severe side-effects. The problem is that the cause of schizophrenia is unknown, and precisely how the drugs affect brain circuitry is also unknown. Schizophrenia is thought to have a substantial environmental component (toxins, culture, upbringing, lifestyle, diet, etc.), but its onset is likely to be predisposed by genetic factors. [1] Genetic analysis has recently made great progress in identifying genes that cause diseases. Many diseases that strike young adults, as schizophrenia often does, have been shown to be caused by one or just a few specific mutations. For example, some diseases that cause blindness are now known to be caused by a mutation in one or more of the genes that code for molecules in the brain essential for sight. In one recent case, gene therapy approved by the FDA to correct the mutation has restored sight in blind people. [2]

Pessimism about schizophrenia
However, research into the possible genetic cause of schizophrenia has not found any obvious candidate gene mutations. Part of the problem is that schizophrenia is not just one disease; it comprises a family of interrelated conditions and is diagnosed by several criteria, which implies that a variety of causes may contribute. Apparently, many gene mutations may contribute to schizophrenia, but none yet found have an influence strong enough to be the exclusive cause. A recent presentation on solving the puzzle of schizophrenia at the Society for Neuroscience (SfN)

conference in Washington DC had a pessimistic tone, explaining that there are no easy answers in the search for better treatment. No helpful novel drug treatments for schizophrenia have been found in recent years, and the lack of obvious genetic markers that are correlated with the disease presents a severe challenge. The SfN presentation, however, didn't mention recent research into dietary causes and treatments for schizophrenia.

Niacin cures many schizophrenics
In the early 1960s, Hoffer and Osmond published studies showing that niacin (also known as nicotinic acid or vitamin B3) given at sufficiently high doses could effectively treat some schizophrenia patients.[3-7] Although Hoffer and Osmond's theories about how niacin could treat schizophrenia were never proven sufficiently to convince the rest of the field, their results in treating thousands of patients with niacin therapy and curing many were striking. The term "orthomolecular" was coined by Linus Pauling for the use of essential nutrients such as niacin in preventing disease, and in particular, schizophrenia.[8] Looking for more recent studies, a search on PubMed of the terms "schizophrenia niacin" returns several dozen articles. One of them asserts that some schizophrenics can be well treated with niacin, and refers to Hoffer and Osmond's early studies, reviewing several theories about likely mechanisms.[9]

"Abram Hoffer backed up his treatment with clearly explained biochemistry, as he had a degree in biochemistry before obtaining his MD. I personally found his presentation fascinating as well as convincing."

(Ralph Campbell, MD)

Niacin skin test
Most people get a "niacin flush" on their skin for a few minutes when a large dose of niacin is taken orally. This is a normal consequence of niacin activating prostaglandin pathways that cause vasodilation in the skin and is not harmful. Niacin is utilized by several hundred metabolic pathways in the body, so oral niacin is taken by many to treat illness and maintain good health.[10] To avoid the skin flush, one starts with small doses [typically 25 mg/day] and gradually increases the dose over several days to achieve a therapeutic effect.[10] However, some schizophrenics don't get a niacin flush with the normal doses, suggesting that they have a deficiency of niacin and likely other essential nutrients. Therefore, niacin applied to the skin or taken orally has been used as a test for predisposition to schizophrenia. Hoffer noted that in some cases where

schizophrenics recovered, they reverted to a normal skin flush.[11] A flurry of recent studies show that about one third of schizophrenics have a blunted niacin skin flush, suggesting that this test can be used as a diagnostic tool. [12-21] Several of these recent studies attempt to determine from those results what aspect of the metabolic disturbance might cause problems for the brain. Although most of these studies don't explicitly discuss the use of niacin as a treatment, the underlying theme is that niacin treatment can help many schizophrenics.[10]

"Dr. Abram Hoffer observed a recovery to a normal niacin-flush response in an otherwise previously flush-resistant schizophrenic. Dr. Hoffer used either niacinamide or niacin, although he favored the lipodystrophy-correcting/flush-causing niacin form more. He also recommended essential fatty acids."

(W. Todd Penberthy, PhD).

Nutrient Dependencies

- Many schizophrenic patients have severe nutrient **dependencies** that can be treated with niacin and other vitamins and nutrients. Several recent studies review the evidence for a benefit from good nutrition (niacin, other B vitamins, vitamin C and D, omega-3 fatty acids, etc.) on brain function. [22-29]
- The use of niacin therapy for testing and treatment of schizophrenia and many other conditions appears to be rapidly expanding. It is inexpensive and widely used for health, but can also help those in desperate need of treatment. For a therapeutic effect, Hoffer recommended gradually increasing doses up to 3,000 mg/day of niacin in divided doses, along with 2,000 mg/day or more of vitamin C and other essential nutrients. For some people, high doses can cause temporary side effects; so many people take niacin for its health benefit at lower doses (500 - 1,000 mg/day). Niacinamide has similar benefits but does not cause the skin flush. For more on the benefits of niacin, dosing, and possible contra-indications please refer to Hoffer's book *"Niacin: the Real Story"* [10].

Conclusion

It is straightforward to understand the historical bias against niacin therapy for schizophrenia. Niacin is inexpensive and can't be patented. And it is known to be effective at preventing heart disease [30]. One can imagine that the drug industry is working to make a form of niacin or a niacin-like drug that can produce profits, [30, 31].

References

- 1. Owen MJ, Sawa A, Mortensen PB. Schizophrenia. Lancet. 2016 Jul 2;388:86-97. https://www.ncbi.nlm.nih.gov/pubmed/26777917
- 2. Ledford H. FDA advisers back gene therapy for rare form of blindness. Nature. 2017 Oct 12;550:314. https://www.nature.com/news/fda-advisers-back-gene-therapy-for-rare-form-of-blindness-1.22819
- 3. Hoffer AF, Osmond H, Smythies, Schizophrenia: a New Approach. II. Results of a Year's Research. J. Mental Sci. 100: 29-45, 1954. https://www.ncbi.nlm.nih.gov/pubmed/13152519
- 4. Hoffer A, Osmond H. Treatment of schizophrenia with nicotinic acid: a ten-year follow-up. Acta Psychiat Scand 1964, 40: 171-189. https://www.ncbi.nlm.nih.gov/pubmed/14235254
- 5. Niacin and Schizophrenia: History and Opportunity. http://orthomolecular.org/resources/omns/v10n18.shtml
- 6. To Give Credit Where Credit is Due. http://orthomolecular.org/resources/omns/v13n05.shtml
- 7. Abram Hoffer Centenary. http://orthomolecular.org/resources/omns/v13n19.shtml
- 8. Pauling L. Orthomolecular psychiatry. Varying the concentrations of substances normally present in the human body may control mental disease. Science. 1968 Apr 19;160:265-271.https://www.ncbi.nlm.nih.gov/pubmed/5641253https://profiles.nlm.nih.gov/ps/access/MMBBJQ.pdf
- 9. Xu XJ, Jiang GS. Niacin-respondent subset of schizophrenia -- a therapeutic review. Eur Rev Med Pharmacol Sci. 2015;19:988-997. https://www.ncbi.nlm.nih.gov/pubmed/25855923
- 10. Hoffer A, Saul AW, Foster HD. Niacin: The Real Story: Learn about the Wonderful Healing Properties of Niacin. Basic Health Publications, Inc; 2015. ISBN-13: 978-1591202752.
- 11. Hoffer A. Adventures in Psychiatry: The Scientific Memoirs of Dr. Abram Hoffer. KOS Publishing, 2005. ISBN-13: 978-0973194562.
- 12. Smesny S, Berger G, Rosburg T, et al. Potential use of the topical niacin skin test in early psychosis -- a combined approach using optical reflection spectroscopy and a descriptive rating scale. Psychiatr Res. 2003 May-Jun;37:237-247. https://www.ncbi.nlm.nih.gov/pubmed/12650743
- 13. Messamore E. Niacin subsensitivity is associated with functional impairment in schizophrenia. Schizophr Res. 2012 May;137(1-3):180-4. https://www.ncbi.nlm.nih.gov/pubmed/22445461
- 14. Lien YJ, Huang SS, Liu CM, et al. A genome-wide quantitative linkage scan of niacin skin flush response in families with schizophrenia. Schizophr Bull. 2013 Jan;39:68-76. https://www.ncbi.nlm.nih.gov/pubmed/21653277
- 15. Nilsson BM, Holm G, Hultman CM, Ekselius L. Cognition and autonomic function in schizophrenia: inferior cognitive test performance in electrodermal and niacin skin flush non-responders. Eur Psychiatry. 2015 Jan;30:8-13. https://www.ncbi.nlm.nih.gov/pubmed/25169443

- 16. Berger GE, Smesny S, Schäfer MR, et al. Niacin Skin Sensitivity Is Increased in Adolescents at Ultra-High Risk for Psychosis. PLoS One. 2016 Feb 19;11(2):e0148429. https://www.ncbi.nlm.nih.gov/pubmed/26894921
- 17. Yao JK, Dougherty GG Jr, Gautier CH, Haas GL, Condray R, Kasckow JW, Kisslinger BL, Gurklis JA, Messamore E. Prevalence and Specificity of the Abnormal Niacin Response: A Potential Endophenotype Marker in Schizophrenia. Schizophr Bull. 2016 Mar;42(2):369-376.https://www.ncbi.nlm.nih.gov/pubmed/26371338
- 18. Sun L, Yang X, Jiang J, et al. Identification of the Niacin-Blunted Subgroup of Schizophrenia Patients from Mood Disorders and Healthy Individuals in Chinese Population. Schizophr Bull. 2017 Oct 25. https://www.ncbi.nlm.nih.gov/pubmed/29077970
- 19. Langbein K, Schmidt U, Schack S, et al. State marker properties of niacin skin sensitivity in ultra-high risk groups for psychosis - An optical reflection spectroscopy study. Schizophr Res. 2017 Jun 8. pii: S0920-9964(17)30335-3. https://www.ncbi.nlm.nih.gov/pubmed/28602647
- 20. Ross BM. Methylnicotinate stimulated prostaglandin synthesis in patients with schizophrenia: A preliminary investigation. Prostaglandins Leukot Essent Fatty Acids. 2017 May 19. pii: S0952-3278(16)30227-7. https://www.ncbi.nlm.nih.gov/pubmed/28552466
- 21. Messamore E. The niacin response biomarker as a schizophrenia endophenotype: A status update. Prostaglandins Leukot Essent Fatty Acids. 2017 Jun 30. pii: S0952-3278(16)30249-6. https://www.ncbi.nlm.nih.gov/pubmed/28688777
- 22. Lim SY, Kim EJ, Kim A, et al. Nutritional Factors Affecting Mental Health. Clin Nutr Res. 2016 Jul; 5:143-52. https://www.ncbi.nlm.nih.gov/pubmed/27482518
- 23. Kim EJ, Lim SY, Lee HJ, et al. Low dietary intake of n-3 fatty acids, niacin, folate, and vitamin C in Korean patients with schizophrenia and the development of dietary guidelines for schizophrenia. Nutr Res. 2017 Sep;45:10-18. https://www.ncbi.nlm.nih.gov/pubmed/29037327
- 24. Pawelczyk T, Piatkowska-Janko E, Bogorodzki P, et al. Omega-3 fatty acid supplementation may prevent loss of gray matter thickness in the left parieto-occipital cortex in first episode schizophrenia: A secondary outcome analysis of the OFFER randomized controlled study. Schizophr Res. 2017 Oct 24. pii: S0920-9964(17)30621-7. https://www.ncbi.nlm.nih.gov/pubmed/29079060
- 25. Marx W, Moseley G, Berk M, Jacka F. Nutritional psychiatry: the present state of the evidence. Proc Nutr Soc. 2017 Nov;76:427-436. https://www.ncbi.nlm.nih.gov/pubmed/28942748
- 26. Cieslak K, Feingold J, Antonius D, et al. Low vitamin D levels predict clinical features of schizophrenia. Schizophr Res. 2014 Nov;159:543-545. https://www.ncbi.nlm.nih.gov/pubmed/25311777 .
- 27. Chiang M, Natarajan R, Fan X. Vitamin D in schizophrenia: a clinical review. Evid Based Ment Health. 2016 Feb;19:6-9. https://www.ncbi.nlm.nih.gov/pubmed/26767392 .
- 28. Akinlade KS, Olaniyan OA, Lasebikan VO, Rahamon SK. Vitamin D Levels in Different Severity Groups of Schizophrenia. Front Psychiatry. 2017 Jun 13;8:105. https://www.ncbi.nlm.nih.gov/pubmed/28659835 .

- 29. Berridge MJ. Vitamin D deficiency: infertility and neurodevelopmental diseases (attention deficit hyperactivity disorder, autism and schizophrenia). Am J Physiol Cell Physiol. 2017 Oct 25:ajpcell.00188.2017. https://www.ncbi.nlm.nih.gov/pubmed/29070492 .
- 30. Goel H, Dunbar RL. Niacin Alternatives for Dyslipidemia: Fool's Gold or Gold Mine? Part II: Novel Niacin Mimetics. Curr Atheroscler Rep. 2016 Apr;18:17. https://www.ncbi.nlm.nih.gov/pubmed/26932224 .
- 31. Dunbar RL, Goel H, Tuteja S, et al. Measuring niacin-associated skin toxicity (NASTy) stigmata along with symptoms to aid development of niacin mimetics. J Lipid Res. 2017 Apr;58:783-797. https://www.ncbi.nlm.nih.gov/pubmed/28119443.

This article may be reprinted free of charge provided 1) that there is clear attribution to the Orthomolecular Medicine News Service, and 2) that both the OMNS free subscription link http://orthomolecular.org/subscribe.html and also the OMNS archive link http://orthomolecular.org/resources/omns/index.shtml are included.

Chapter IVX: Quotes from Famous Historical Vegetarians:

"Nothing will benefit human health and increase the chances of survival of life as much as the evolution to a vegetarian diet." --Albert Einstein 1879-1955.

"The average age of a meat eater is 63. I am on the verge of 85 and still work as hard as ever. I have lived quite long enough and I am trying to die, but I simply cannot do it. A single beef steak would finish me; but I cannot bring myself to swallow it. I am oppressed with the dread of living forever. That is the only disadvantage to vegetarianism," --George Bernard Shaw, prior to his 85th birthday.

"I have, from an early age, abjured the use of meat, and the time will come when men such as I will look on the murder of animals as they now look on the murder of men." -Leonardo Da Vinci 1452-1519.

"Whenever I injure any kind of life, I must be quite certain that it is necessary. I must never go beyond the unavoidable, not ever in apparently insignificant things. That man is truly ethical who shatters no ice crystal as it sparkles in the sun, tears no leaf from a tree." --Albert Schweitzer.

In 1968 one of the great minds of the 20st. Century, two time Nobel Prize winner Linus Pauling, Ph. D, coined the term Orthomolecular

Nutrition. "Orthomolecular" is, literally, "pertaining to the right molecule." Dr. Pauling proposed that by giving the body the right molecules (optimum nutrition) most disease would be eradicated. He went on to say, *"Every element, every sickness, and every disease can be traced back to an organic trace mineral deficiency."* (Categorical statement).

To substantiate Linus Pauling's statement, I quote *"It is a fact that 99% of Americans are deficient in organic minerals because 'inorganic (i.e., toxic, synthetic, dead, and inert) chemicals, pesticides, and herbicides have destroyed nearly all the critical organic complexes, elements, and minerals in our soils."* 74th. Congress, second session regarding organic minerals (categorical statement).

Remember Dr. Robert H. Fletcher M.D. and Kathleen M. Fairfield, M.D., Ph. D. study results, *"Their findings definitively confirm that all diseases find their roots in nutritive poor and specifically poor mineral nutrition. This lack of minerals in the body manifests itself as diseases."*

C. Everett Koop, M.D., Sc. D, former two times Surgeon General of the United States, produced the first Surgeon General's Report on Nutrition and Health in 1988. It was based on an exhaustive review of the scientific literature. He concluded that "dietary excess and imbalance" contributed significantly to eight of the leading killer diseases in the United States. Dr. Koop highlighted six areas where dietary excess and imbalance were contributing factors in death:

1. Diet has a vital influence on health.
2. Five of the ten leading causes of illness and death are associated with diet (coronary heart disease, cancer, stroke, diabetes and atherosclerosis).
3. Another three have been associated with excessive alcohol intake (cirrhosis of the liver, accidents, and suicide).
4. These eight conditions accounted for nearly 1.5 million of the 2.1 million total deaths in 1987.
5. Dietary excesses or imbalances also contribute to other problems such as high blood pressure, obesity, dental diseases, osteoporosis, and gastrointestinal diseases.
6. It is now clear that diet contributes in substantial ways to the development of these diseases and that modification of diet can contribute to their prevention and control.

Just to drive the point home, I will quote another credible source. The World Health Organization (WHO) commissioned a panel of nutrition experts from around the world. The result, a 200–page technical paper titled, "Diet, Nutrition and the Prevention of Chronic Diseases," was published in 1990. In addition, an executive summary was published in 1991. It concluded: Medical and scientific research has established clear links between dietary factors and the risk of developing coronary artery disease, hypertension stroke, several cancers, osteoporosis, diabetes, and other chronic disease.

Finally, I will share the information produced during the China Study. Drawing on the project's findings in rural China, but going far beyond those findings, the China Study details the connection between nutrition and heart disease, diabetes and cancer. The report also examines the source of nutritional confusion produced by powerful lobbies, government entities, and opportunistic scientists. The New York Times has recognized the study (China-Oxford-Cornell Diet and Health Project) as the "Grand Prix of epidemiology" and the "most comprehensive large study ever undertaken of the relationship between diet and the risk of developing disease."

In 1995, Time magazine introduced the world to phyto-chemicals. Today, more than 100,000 such disease fighting nutrients have been discovered in fruits and vegetables. Agriculture, especially organic farming, is an integral component of the wellness program. Fruits and vegetables are loaded with compounds called phytochemicals and antioxidants that demonstrably lower the risk of cancer and fight other diseases. As few as twenty years ago, you could discount the diet and nutrition link to optimal mental and physical health, but today with all the scientific data available, one will only hasten their death by ignoring it.

Chapter XV: Case Studies

A young man age 15 at the time was referred to me by his Psychiatrist, in September of 2016. He was previously hospitalized at Nicklaus Children's Hospital in Miami, Florida and was discharged April 14, 2016 with a diagnose of "unspecified psychosis". He was prescribed acetaminophen, diphenhydramine injection, immune globulin intravenous, and nystatin. His as need medication was epinephrine injection, Benadryl injection, and methylprednisolone injection. According to his mother, he had been on nine different psychotic drugs over a two year period.

When his mother brought the young man to his first appointment, he was very non-coherent, lack of attention or focus, very uninterested and zombie like. His mother had to direct his every movement. As with all my patients, I did a body chemistry analysis, which is based upon the Reams Biological Theory of Ionization (RBTI). The purpose of RBTI is to analyze and identify previously unrecognized electro-biochemical

dysfunctions taking place within the human body, thereby allowing the creation of a perfect set of personal life-style recommendations that will address and reverse those unrecognized dysfunctional patterns. His numbers (analysis results) were very interesting in that there were several concerns that had to be resolved in my mind before a specific diagnosis could be determined, if one was really warranted. The fact that he was diagnosed with 'unspecified psychosis' added validity to the RBTI as a tool for screening for mental disease along with other tests and lab work. His RBTI results showed that his blood sugar and salt levels were way above the normal range causing a decreased supply of oxygen to the brain. His pH was acid and his urea numbers were too high and both were compounding his mental health problems. He was extremely
Dehydrated, so I immediately instructed the mother to take her child to the hospital emergency room and wrote an order for an intravenous (I.V.) of fluid. When the mother brought the young man back for his next appointment she stated that she "can get him to do anything she wants when he is hydrated but three or four days after the IV, he begins to deteriorate." The patient said that he does not want to drink water, so I explained the importance of hydration and the brain to him and his mother. I advised his mother that the next time he does an IV to do a half-dose (half the sodium) because his salts were already too high. The mother wanted me to write another order for a I.V. treatment for her son, so I did.

    As we continued the appointment, we discussed his diet; parent said that he eats only junk food. When I asked if they keep junk food in the house, the mother and grandmother looked at each other and started laughing, admitting that they eat junk foods as well. The patient said that he wants to starve to death than eat the food his mother prepares. His mother says that he rummages through the kitchen at night, which tells her that he wants to eat. I explained to both of them how critical it was for him to eat a good and nutritious diet and it's affects upon the brain. We discussed his digestive system and his mother felt that he has parasites, which I addressed.

    Several days later after his second I.V. treatment the mother called the clinic and said that her son was back to normal again and was pleasant and doing fine in school. A few more days passed and the mother called again wanting me to write an order for another I.V. I instructed the mother that this was going to be the last order that I write if they do not start implementing the program and diet that I had wrote up for him to follow. I explained to her that it was time to parent, showing him tough love if necessary. I explained to her that she and her mother had to be the example for their son. She had to remove all junk food from her home and if she wanted to eat it that was her choice but not in front of her son. That they needed to drink more water in front of him and encourage him to drink with them. Basically, I emphasized that they had to do the program along with him and not expect a fifteen year old to make these difficult changes by himself. He was allowed to develop these habits over the years and he needs support and leadership.

Several days later the mother called me again with information I was already anticipating. While at the hospital, a nurse was giving her a difficult time about giving the young man another I.V. The nurse did not believe that the I.Vs. were working. The mother then told me that she asked the nurse to explain then how her son returns to normal after an I.V., which the nurse could not answer. The nurse observed the child's behavior twice now when he first came in to be treated and observed his behavior immediately after the I.V. and was unable to explain the drastic change. Remember the study under Dr. water entitled brain serotonin metabolism during water deprivation and hydration in rats? This study helps to explain this young man's behavior and the need for a nutritional profile before a person, especially the youth are given damaging psychotropic drugs. I once again reiterated to the mother that she needed to parent and start making changes or her only other option was to put him back on the psychotropic drugs.

The mother emailed me about six months later asking me to work with her son again. I stated to her that he needs to be willing to make the necessary changes I recommended or I would not be of any value to him. I asked her to specifically ask him if he was ready to make those changes. To date, I have not heard back from the mother.

In my twenty-year career as a Naturopath, I have worked with patients with bio-polar, mild to medium depression, anxiety, etc. and after doing the RBTI analysis' on them, I can count the number of patients on one hand that I had to refer to a psychiatrist. When a person is committed to following the program outlined it is a joy to me and God to see broken hearts mended, families finding the fun of living, new goals set and achieved, barriers to growth and fulfillment torn down, new direction to new horizons--these are only a few of the exciting rewards that come from implementing the principles of God's
Ten Doctors and trusting Him with the results.

Case Study #2
While writing this book in 2018, a mother brought her 29 year old son to the clinic that had recently been diagnosed with Schizophreniform illness with catatonic features. The young man had gone to college on a track

scholarship and was in good physical condition. She stated that a person at her son's place of employment had referred her son to me and wanted to know if I could help. His current medication included: clonazepam, 2mg; lactulose, 15 mL; lorazepam, 2 mg; Metoprolol Succinate 50mg; Risperidone 1mg; Mirtazapine 15mg; Benztropine 2mg; and Olanzapine, 5mg. After listening to the patient's mother recite his recent health history, I did a body chemistry analysis. The analysis results revealed that his numbers were almost normal except in for his immune system and his digestive system. I asked the patient for a copy of his most recent lab results. The next day, the patient's mother stopped by the clinic and handed to me 51 pages of Emergency Physician Notes, Mental Health Notes, Haematology, INR Reference Range, Chemistry, Serology, Urine Studies, Reference Laboratory Reports, Microbiology, Magentic Rasonance Imaging, and Radiology. After reviewing fifty-one pages of reports and my own analysis it became crystal clear that the your man's biggest problem was his

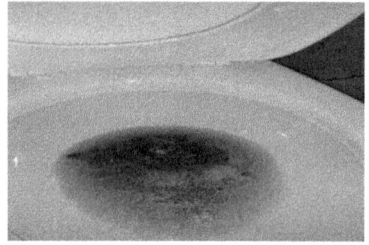

digestive system, especially his colon. He may have a mild form of schizophrenia, but until his digestive issues were resolved, it is premature to treat him with such strong psychotropic (mind altering) drugs. On the next visit the patient's father attended along with the patient and his mother. The mother wanted her son off the prescription medication because she felt it was making him feel and behave worse, while the dad was not opposed to taking his son off the medication but wanted to know what could be done for him naturally. I explained and showed him studies of nutritional and herbal approaches to healing mental disease. He agreed to support his son and take the natural approach to his mental health. I gave the patient Gota Kola for cognitive function, ginseng for body alertness, St. John's wort for his depression, valerian root for anxiety brought on by depression and gingko biloba as Researchers believe that ginkgo improves cognitive function because it promotes good blood circulation in the brain and protects the brain and other parts from neuronal damage. As well as 5-HTP which facilitates the metabolic process in the serotonin brain cell's manufacturing process, also provided patient with a program to follow, which included vitamins and minerals; and a plant based menu of nutrient dense foods.

The mother took him off all psychotropic drugs without my knowledge. I explained my concerns of being so constipated and the strong psychotic drugs in his system, and what I knew should happen before he is labeled with a mental health condition. I needed to know if his constipation started first or did his strange behaviors manifest first. Because according to the analysis I performed, his digestive enzymes were very acidic, which meant he should be been suffering from diarrhea but instead was constipated. His mother stated that every since he started taking the prescription drugs, he started getting worse, e.g. behavior, constipation, lack of appetite, etc… I place the patient on a three-day cleanse and detoxification program. On the first day of the program, while giving a colon irrigation treatment the largest mass of hard stool came out of this young man. The pictures above show the specimen; it was 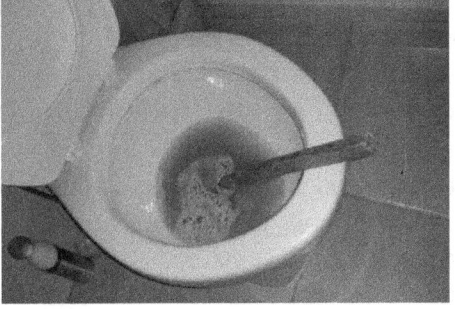 so large and hard that it could not be flushed down the toilet. It took a hard stick and several minutes of pounding to break it up before it could be flushed down the toilet. The mother reported that after the colon irrigation her son was responding positively in every way and improving slowly. It is still too soon to know if her son truly has a mental disease, so we shall allow the process of symptoms, behavior; test results and the patient's own assessment of himself determine which direction his treatment plan goes. After several days the patient started to regress almost to the point where he was when he first came to see me. After doing another body chemistry analysis, I increased his nutrient in take to support his immune system. I called an acquaintance of mine, a medical doctor at a different hospital that agreed to see him. After examining him, the doctor questioned why he was on high blood pressure medication when he didn't have high blood pressure then rescheduled another appointment because he saw him on short notice. A few days later, while my M.D. friend was away his mother brought the patient into the clinic to show me that over the weekend he started bleeding and his mouth and teeth were covered with blood. I immediately advised her to take him to the emergency room at the hospital. She was reluctant to because she felt that the hospital had misdiagnosed him from the beginning. So I had her take him to the hospital were my friend work.

    These heart wrenching events took place in less than three months time. The hospital that my M.D. friend worked at transferred the patient by ambulance because they do not have an emergency department, to the hospital that had misdiagnosed him and they continued to treat him for Schizophrenia. To make a long and sad story short, I had him transferred out of that hospital to third hospital. They immediately put him in the Intensive Care Unit (ICU) and assigned a hematologist and internist to his case. The young man died shortly thereafter from Lupus! As you know Lupus is a systemic autoimmune disease that occurs when your body's immune system attacks your own tissues and organs. Inflammation caused by lupus can affect many different body systems — including your joints, skin, kidneys, blood cells, **brain**, heart and lungs. Many diseases like Lupus affects body organs like the brain and that is why psychotic drugs should be the last option and not the first. In looking back over this young man's medical records for the previous year, it was clear that so many misfortunate turn of events took place, some even on his part that lead to this tragic ending. If the medical doctors would have considered what the mother was saying because she knew her son, they had a special relationship.

Even at the late stage that his mother brought him to me, if the medical doctors had of considered my findings and test recommendations this young man might be alive today. Once again I strongly encourage people to consider all the symptoms and conditions that could be causing abnormal behavior like constipation, poor nutrition, a lack of proper water intake, etc... before accepting a diagnoses of chemical imbalance of the brain, for which no scientific medical test can detect or confirm and start taking psychotropic drugs.

Chapter XVI: Safety of Natural Healing vs. Synthetic Chemicals

To entertain this false argument is to give it validity. If you read the side effects of Prozac, Paxcel, Zolfoft, etc... Concerning Prozac you are warned "Prozac side effects... "Report any new or worsening symptoms to your doctor, such as: mood or behavior changes, anxiety, panic attacks, trouble sleeping, or if you feel impulsive, irritable, agitated, hostile, aggressive, restless, hyperactive (mentally or physically), more depressed, or have thoughts about suicide or hurting yourself or others. The mind is a very delicate organ and antidepressants can influence it to do evil as well as assist it to avoid
hurting its host. We also read earlier that antidepressants have the opposite affect after prolonged use, as well as SSRI does not increase the level of serotonin in the blood. Yes, there is the possibility of someone hurting themselves or someone else because a diagnosis was missed, like in the medical profession. Or a person does not completely follow their

program, just like to person not taking their prescription medication in the medical profession.
- However did you know that there are no population control studies to determine the synergism of using multiple drugs.
- "The National Institute of Health (NIH), which is in Bethesda, Maryland, near the capitol of the US, is arguably, the most advanced medical research unit in the world. It has been in existence for a hundred years. It has 18,000 employees, thousands of medical researchers and over the last hundred years it has received from the taxpayer's pockets (of Americans), hard-working taxpayers, over a trillion dollars. In that hundred years and thousands of researchers and over a trillion dollars in research funded it has not found the cure for one single disease, ever."
--Dr. Lorraine Day, MD, Acclaimed Orthopedic Trauma Surgeon, 20-yr breast cancer survivor and Best-selling author. (excerpt taken from her interview on the Russell Scott radio show).
- Also, did you know that The FDA and mainstream media have been taunting for several years now that taking vitamins, minerals, and supplements are dangerous. Statistics prove otherwise. According to a 251-page report from the U.S. National Poison Data System the number of people killed in 2014 across America by vitamins, minerals, amino acids or herbal supplements is exactly zero.

FOR IMMEDIATE RELEASE
Orthomolecular Medicine News Service, January 5, 2017
No Deaths from Supplements. No Deaths from Minerals or Amino Acids. No Deaths from Homeopathics or Herbs.
By Andrew W. Saul, Editor

(OMNS, Jan 5, 2017) Not only are there no deaths from vitamins, there are also **zero deaths from *any* supplement**. The most recent (2015) information collected by the U.S. National Poison Data System, and published in the journal Clinical Toxicology (1), shows no deaths whatsoever from dietary supplements.

No deaths from minerals
There were zero deaths from any dietary mineral supplement. This means there were no fatalities from calcium, magnesium, chromium, zinc, colloidal silver, selenium, iron, or multimineral supplements. Reported in the "Electrolyte and Mineral" category was a fatality from the medical use of "Sodium and sodium salts" and another fatality from non-supplemental iron, which was clearly and specifically excluded from the supplement category.

No deaths from any other nutritional supplement
Additionally, there were zero deaths from any amino acid or herbal product. This means no deaths at all from blue cohosh, echinacea, ginkgo biloba, ginseng, kava kava,[St. John's wort], valerian, yohimbe, Asian medicines, ayurvedic medicines, or any other botanical. There were zero deaths from creatine, blue-green algae, glucosamine, chondroitin, or melatonin. There were zero deaths from any homeopathic remedy.

But when in doubt, blame a supplement. Any supplement.
There actually was one fatality alleged from some "Unknown Dietary Supplement or Homeopathic Agent." This is hearsay at best, and scaremongering at worst. How can an accusation be based on the unknown? Claiming causation without even knowing what substance or ingredient to accuse is baseless.

The truth: no man, woman or child died from any nutritional supplement. Period!
If nutritional supplements are allegedly so "dangerous," as the FDA, the news media, and even some physicians still claim, then *where are the bodies*?

References:
Mowry JB, Spyker DA, Brooks DE et al. 2015 Annual Report of the American Association of Poison Control Centers' National Poison Data System (NPDS): 33rd Annual Report. *Clinical Toxicology 2016*, 54:10, 924-1109, http://dx.doi.org/10.1080/15563650.2016.1245421

Data for minerals, herbs, amino acids, and other supplements are presented in Table 22-B.

The complete 187-page article is available for free download from https://aapcc.s3.amazonaws.com/pdfs/annual_reports/2015_AAPCC_NPDS_Annual_Report_33rd_PDF.pdfor download this and all previous AAPCC Annual Reports at http://www.aapcc.org/annual-reports/

- This article may be reprinted free of charge provided 1) that there is clear attribution to the Orthomolecular Medicine News Service, and 2) that both the OMNS free subscription link http://orthomolecular.org/subscribe.html and also the OMNS archive link http://orthomolecular.org/resources/omns/index.shtml are included.

The public have the right to be fully informed as to the benefits and risk of either approach, so they can make an intelligent decision. We need a level playing field by not banning natural substances like L-Tryptophan that can only be given by a prescription, which most medical doctors and psychiatrist will not do. The public has to know that it is available and the benefits of using it in order to be able to make an informed decision. No the issue is not that a misdiagnoses might be made or that someone might not follow their program completely, but rather the millions of dollars lost in revenues and share holders profits.

In contrast, few people connect antidepressant drugs with the acts of violent crimes. Case in point, the recent school shooting in Florida, was perpetrated by an individual with a history of mental disease. Which antidepressant(s) was he on? Did he stop taking them? This information is left out of the mainstream Medias broadcast and the focus is diverted to gun control! The real culprit is the Pharmeuctical industry and those who uphold the system of poisoning peoples' frontal lobe and the brain.

School Shootings & Violence
In 2007 I quit keeping track but one thing is clear, every single incident the individual(s) were on or recently on antidepressant drugs.

Blackburg, VA, April 16, 2007: Seung-Hui Cho went on a rampage of violence that ended with 33 dead and more than two dozen injured, making it the most deadly shooting spree in American history. Antidepressants were found among his belongings.

Littleton, CO, April 20, 1999: Eric Harris and Dylan Klebold, armed with knives, guns, and bombs, terrorized Columbine High School, killing 13 and wounding 23 before shooting themselves. Harris was taking Luvox.

Red Lake Indian Reservation, MN, March 21, 2005: Jeffery Weise killed his grandfather and his grandfather's girlfriend, then went to Red Lake High School where he killed seven more people and wounded more than a dozen others before taking his own life. He was taking Prozac.

Springfield, OR, May 21, 1998: Kip Kinkel murdered his parents, and then proceeded to school where he killed two students and wounded more than 20 more. He was taking Prozac.

Bailey, CO, September 27, 2006: Duane Morrison went into Platte Canyon High School and took six teenage girls hostage, sexually assaulting some of them and shooting one in the head before killing himself. Antidepressant medication was found in his jeep.

Violence in the Workplace
Louisville, KY, September 14, 1989: Joseph Wesbecker marched into work with an AK-47 and other guns, killed eight employees, wounded 12, and committed suicide. He was taking Prozac.

Wakefield, MA, December 26, 2000: Michael McDermott gunned down seven of his colleagues at Edgewater Technology. He was taking Prozac.

Meridian, MS, July 8, 2003: Doug Williams opened fire on coworkers at Lockheed Martin with a 12-gauge shotgun, killing five and injuring nine others before taking his own life. He was taking Zoloft and Celexa.

Newington, CT, March 6, 1998: Disgruntled lottery accountant Matthew Beck killed four colleagues before fatally shooting himself. He was taking Luvox.

Royal Oak, MI, November 14, 1991: Ex-postal employee Thomas McIlvane shot nine people, killing three, at his former place of business before shooting himself in the head. He was taking Prozac.

Stoughton, MA, August 5, 1997: Richard Shurman fatally shot two of his business partners. He was taking Zoloft.

Brutal Murders
Huntsville, AL, March 10, 1998: Jeffery Franklin killed both of his parents with a hatchet and attempted to murder three of his younger siblings. He was taking Ritalin, Prozac, and Klonopin.

Purcell, OK, April 12, 2006: Kevin Underwood murdered and sexually assaulted a 10-year-old girl. Authorities said he had plans for cannibalism. He was taking Lexapro.

Augusta, MT, August 26, 2002: Jeanette Swanson shot and killed her two youngest children while they slept. She was taking Paxil.

Bosie, ID, September 2, 2003: Sarah Johnson shot and killed both of her parents, allegedly because they did not approve of the boy she was dating. She was taking Zoloft.

Wakefield, MA, January 10, 2001: Previously mild-mannered 81-year-old Anthony Dalesando repeatedly stabbed his wife of nearly 50 years with a kitchen knife while she slept. He was taking several medications including Prozac.

Alamogordo, NM, July 5, 2004: Fourteen-year-old Cody Posey killed his father, stepmother, and stepsister. He then hid the bodies and broke a window with an ax to suggest an intruder had committed the murders. He was taking Zoloft.

Dr. Abram Hoffer said it best ""<u>For schizophrenia, the recovery rate with drug therapy is under 15%. With nutritional therapy, the recovery rate is 80%.</u>" --<u>Dr. Abram Hoffer **M.D.**</u>

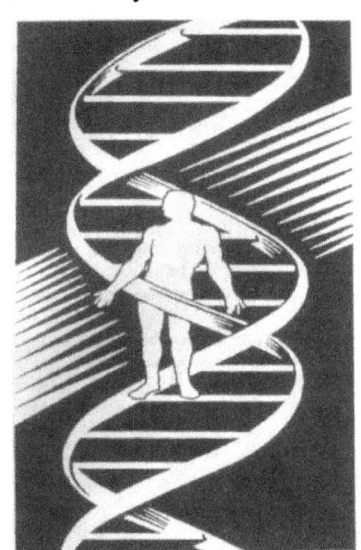

Does the pharmaceutical industry and those who benefit and profit from them really care about human life, or are they more concerned that you are not taking their antidepressants? Undoubtedly, one has to know when to refer a patient for more intense psychiatric care. Psychiatrist, medical doctors, the American Medical Association and American Psychiatrist Association as well need to recognize and acknowledge the rightful place Orthomolecular Nutrition plays in the healing process; and not place patients on antidepressants the first visit; specifically if they are not harmful to themselves or to others, then refer them out for a Reams Biological Theory of Ionization (RBTI) analysis and work with the Naturopathic doctor that knows and understands RBTI and therapeutic nutrition.

Make A New You Physically & Spiritually: John 3:3
"Health is a matter of choice, not a mystery of chance." -Robert A. Mendelsohn, M.D.

Remember, as I have already stated in an earlier chapter, God has created the body to heal itself. Relying and depending on man's pharmaceuticals do more harm than good in the long run, and interferes with this innate healing process. Trust God and find a competent Christian Health Practitioner that believes in and practices God's Ten Doctors and patiently work with your body and it will heal. The only time, and I repeat the only time allopathic intervention is necessary or required is when a person become a potential harm to them self or someone else.
God has sent you his word in this book and can heal you, and deliver you from destruction (antidepressants), based on Psalms 107:20.

James says, *"But let patience have [her] perfect work, that ye may be perfect and entire, wanting nothing"* James 1:4. It takes time to heal as the above information points out, but we have been programmed to want instant relief at whatever the cost.

The word of God says that "Men's hearts (minds) failing them for fear..." Luke 21:26. If you want the peace and tranquility of mind God has promised "Thou wilt keep *him* in perfect peace, *whose* mind *is* stayed *on thee:* because he trusteth in thee. Trust ye in the LORD for ever: for in the LORD JEHOVAH *is* everlasting strength" Isa. 26: 3, 4.

Maranatha,
office@originalhealing.org

References & End Notes: the second number corresponds with Dr. Chalmers book, Healing the Broken Brain.

1/64 Achterberg & Lawlis, Bridges of the Bodymind. Champaign, IL: Institute Personality & Ability Testing, 1980.
2/65 Borysenko, Joan. Minding the Body, Mending the Mind.. Reading, Mass. Addison-Wesley Publishing Company, Inc. 1987
3/66 Wenzlaff, Richard "The Mental Control of Depression," in Wenger and Pennebaker, Handbook of Mental Control.
4/67 Beck, Aaron. Love is Never Enough. New York: Harper and Row, 1988, pg. 145-146.
5/68 KJV Bible book of Matthew, chapter 9, verse 6.
6/69 KJV Bible book of Hebrews, chapter 11, verse 1.
7/70 KJV Bible book of Romans, chapter 10, verse 17.
8/71 KJV Bible book of 1 John, chapter 5, verse 18.
9/72 KJV Bible book of 1 Corinthians, chapter 13, verses 4-7.
10/73 KJV Bible book of Philippians, chapter 3, verse 13.
11/74 KJV Bible book of Galatians, chapter 6, verse 7.
12/75 White, Steps to Christ, p. 57, 58.
13/102 KJV Bible book of Isaiah, chapter 58, verse 1.
14/103 KJV Bible book of Isaiah, chapter 40, verses 1, 2.
15/104 KJV Bible book of John, chapter 16, verse 12.
16/105 KJV Bible book of I Corinthians, chapter 9, verse 25.
17/108 Davis, C. M. Self-selection of diet by newly weaned infants. *American Journal of Diseases of Children*, 1928, 36, 651-679.
18/109 Richter, C., and Eckert, J.F. Mineral metabolism of adrenalectomized rats studied by the appetite method. *Endocrinology,* 1938, 22, 214-224.
19/110 Chalmers, Elden M. Unpublished study done at the university of Tennessee, 1967.

20/111 Wilkins, L. and Richter, C. P. A. A great craving for salt by a child with cortico-adrenal insufficiency. *Journal of the American Medical Association*, 1940, 114, 866-868.

21/112 KJV Bible book of Matthews, chapter 25, verses 14-30.

22/113 White, E.G. Education, Mt. View, CA: Pacific Press Assn, 1903, p. 29.

23/114 Kegan, R. G. (1986). The child behind the mask: Sociopathy as developmental delay. In W. W. Reid, D. Dorr, J.I. Walker, & J.W. Benner III (Eds.), Unmasking the psychopath, p. 45-77, New York: W. W. Norton.

24/115 Magid, Ken & McKelvey, Carole A. 1987. High Risk, Children without a Conscience, New York: Bantam Books 1989

White, Ellen. Acts of the Apostles (AA)
Pacific Press Publishing Association, Mountain View, California. 1911.

White, Ellen. Adventist Home (AH)
Review and Herald Publishing Association, Washington, D.C. 1952.

White, Ellen. Council on Diet and Foods (CDF)
Review and Herald Publishing Association, Washington, D.C. 1938.

White, Ellen. Christ Object Lessons: (COL)
Review and Herald Publishing Association, Washington, D.C. 1900.

White, Ellen. Desire of Ages: (DA)
Pacific Press Publishing Association, Mountain View, California, 1940.

White, Ellen. Fundamentals of Christian Education
Southern Publishing Association, Nashville, TN 1923.

White, Ellen. The Great Controversy (GC)
Pacific Press Publishing Association, Mountain View, Calif. 1888 and 1911.

White, Ellen. Medical Ministry
Pacific Press Publishing Association, Mountain View, Calif. 1932.

White, Ellen. Messages to Young People (MYP)
>Review & Herald Publishing Association, Washington, D.C. 1930.

White, Ellen. My Life Today (ML)
>Review & Herald Publishing Association, Washington, D.C. 1952.

White, Ellen. Patriarchs and Prophets (PP)
>Review & Herald Publishing Association, Washington, D.C. 1890.

>Review and Herald (RH), Aug. 8. 1894
>Review & Herald Publishing Association, Washington, D.C.

White, Ellen. Selected Messages, Book 1 (1SM)
>Pacific Press Publishing Association, Mountain View, Calif. 1958.

White, Ellen. Selected Messages, Book 2 (2SM)
>Review & Herald Publishing Association, Washington, D.C., 1958.

White, Ellen. Seventh-day Adventist Bible Commentary (SDABC), vol. 7, p. 977.

White, Ellen. Steps to Christ (SC)
>Pacific Press Publishing Association, Mountain View, California. 1892.

Temperance (Te)
>Pacific Press Publishing Association, Mountain View, Calif., 1949.

White, Ellen. Testimonies for the Church, Vol. 5 (2T)
>Pacific Press Publishing Association, Mountain View, Calif. 1871.

White, Ellen. Testimonies for the Church, Vol. 5 (4T)

Pacific Press Publishing Association, Mountain View, Calif. 1881.

White, Ellen. <u>Testimonies for the Church, Vol. 5</u> (5T)
Pacific Press Publishing Association, Mountain View, Calif. 1889.

White, Ellen. <u>Testimonies to Ministers</u> (TM)
Pacific Press Publishing Association, Mountain View, Calif. 1923.

White, Ellen. <u>Thoughts from the Mount of Blessings</u> (TMB)
Pacific Press Publishing Association, Mountain View, Calif. 1896.

www.ingramcontent.com/pod-product-compliance
Lightning Source LLC
Chambersburg PA
CBHW070144230526
45471CB00002B/513